THE THRI

G000065514

A WOMAN'S GUIDE TO

THRIVING

AFTER

PROSTATE CANCER

You've Helped Him Through —
Now What About You?

CINDIE HUBIAK

FOREWORD BY LARRY L. BANS, MD,
MEDICAL DIRECTOR, PROSTATE SOLUTIONS OF ARIZONA

For permission and reprint information, contact:
Applied Synergistcs International, Inc.
P.O. Box 5737, Scottsdale, AZ 85261
info@SolutionsForIntimacy

Disclaimer

The author of this book does not dispense medical advice or prescribe the use of any technique as a form of treatment. All matters pertaining to your mental and physical health should be supervised by a health care provider. The author and publisher shall have neither liability nor responsibility to any person or entity with respect to any loss, damage, or injury caused, directly or indirectly, by the use of the information contained in this book.

Library of Congress Control Number: 2011912305

Hubiak, Cindie
    A woman's guide to thriving after prostate cancer : you've helped him through—now what about you? / Cindie Hubiak—1st ed.
        ISBN: 978-0-9837913-0-0
        1. Hubiak, Cindie—Health 2. Prostate—Cancer 3. Sex 4. Prostate—Cancer—Complications 5. Impotence 6. Prostate—Cancer—Family relationships 7. Women 8. Personal Growth

Editor: Barbara McNichol Editorial
Cover and Interior Design: 1106 Design
Photo of Cindie Hubiak: Julie Boles

Printed in the U.S.A.

DEDICATION

I dedicate this book to my husband, Steve Frohman,
who, after recovering from prostate cancer, continues to help
me learn new ways to thrive. I also dedicate this book to
all the teachers who assisted me along the way.

TABLE OF CONTENTS

FOREWORD

AS A UROLOGIST WHO treats men with prostate cancer, I focus on their physical well-being while also being acutely sensitive to their emotional state. Specifically, my experience shows that physicians tend to focus mostly on the physical aspects of erectile function. But an important piece of the healing journey often gets overlooked in the prostate cancer story—the physical and emotional well-being of a patient's spouse. Yet this person plays a huge part in surviving the challenges every couple faces.

My eyes have been opened to this dimension, thanks to my patient Steve's wife Cindie, who has candidly written this book for fellow female cancer survivors. *A Woman's Guide to Thriving after Prostate Cancer: You've Helped Him Through—Now What About You?* offers more than an eye-opening experience. It shows how to apply concrete ideas and practices to a woman's own odyssey through her loved one's prostate cancer journey.

This guide fills in potentially ruinous gaps that couples—and medical professionals—can miss when addressing all aspects of prostate cancer. Cindie has turned the spotlight on what women (including caregivers, friends, and close relatives) need to know about their own emotional well-being. Indeed, she takes the issue to a whole new level as she ties sensuality and intimacy into sexuality with the goal of enhancing a couples' experience. Following her suggestions can help both women and men avoid needless pain and hasten their healing. Perhaps the biggest benefit of all is learning to actually *thrive*—sex life and all—after prostate cancer.

Within the pages of *A Woman's Guide to Thriving after Prostate Cancer,* may you find inspiration to face your healing journey with the kind of courage and newfound confidence Cindie exemplifies. May you use her suggestions so you, too, can make the momentous changes you want in your intimate relationship. And may you take your vitality for living in this world to a whole new dimension.

A Woman's Guide to Thriving after Prostate Cancer points you in the right direction.

Larry L. Bans, MD
Medical Director
Prostate Solutions of Arizona
Phoenix, Arizona

My Prostate Cancer Journey—and Yours

MANY PEOPLE BELIEVE the topic of surviving prostate cancer relates only to men. It doesn't. This disease can take a serious toll on women, too. Its impact depends on the woman's relationship with the man diagnosed with this type of cancer. Whether she's his wife, lover, mother, sister, daughter, friend, or colleague, there's an impact on her life.

I wrote this book primarily for women living in survival mode in the aftermath of their man's prostate cancer. I wrote it for women like the one who told me she and her husband divorced after 16 years of marriage because of the isolation it caused. And I wrote it for women like me who want to learn how to *thrive* when their lives are upended because of the prostate cancer experience.

That said, *any* woman can gain insights into creating a thriving life—sex life included—from my journey of self-discovery. So can men who've been diagnosed with prostate cancer. It helps them more fully understand what their women experience and provides ways to participate in their shift from *surviving* to *thriving*.

My own experience began when my husband, Steve, first heard the words "you have prostate cancer." Like many men, he didn't want anyone to know. So for three years, I honored his request to keep his diagnosis and surgery private. Finding it extremely tough not to tell others, I suffered because of my silence. I hated hiding something so significant in my life. I felt like a hypocrite.

Over time, with Steve's agreement, I shared his situation with a few people, but none of them was in the same situation. Yes, it helped to have them listen, yet I was often too embarrassed to talk about my own predicament. Thinking no one could understand or help me, I didn't want to burden them with how miserable my life had become.

Despite my continual search, I couldn't find any resources that specifically addressed a woman's situation after her man was diagnosed with prostate cancer. I found a lot of information for men and some for couples, but specific resources for women weren't apparent or easy to find. After all, *we* women didn't receive the cancer diagnosis, and *our* bodies weren't directly affected.

Naturally, all the attention focused on the men—a rationale that made sense to me. In fact, Steve and I did exactly that: we directed all our attention toward him. Making sure he lived a cancer-free life became our top priority and rightly so—at least at first.

Yet my life simply didn't work after his diagnosis. So I started searching for ways to "fix" Steve and to "fix" us. After a year or so, I discovered this: When I centered on *my own recovery process*—voila—answers showed up in a variety of places and through many people.

Today, I live a thriving, fulfilling life *despite* our prostate cancer experience . . . or maybe *because* of it!

In part because of all I learned on my journey, Steve made a surprising choice last year. He has transitioned his consulting business from working with organizations to focusing on individuals. Today, instead of hiding, Steve now directs a team of professionals who assist men and couples to live a fulfilling life after prostate cancer—sex and all!

My silence is over. Our friends, relatives, and colleagues know I not only survived prostate cancer but also moved beyond surviving to *thriving*.

Because of my outreach, I met a number of men and women whose lives were deeply affected by this cancer. I talked with sisters, sisters-in-law, professional contacts, and daughters. I answered questions from men who have recovered from treatment, and I spoke with newly diagnosed men as well as those striving to keep their prostates healthy.

I've learned that, yes, women too can survive prostate cancer and become healthier and happier after the experience. This journey wasn't easy for me. I made mistakes and took too many detours along the way. But four years after Steve's diagnosis, I finally live a life I love!

I hope this guide helps you avoid pain and hasten your healing by learning from my journey. It's my intention that you find inspiration, fresh ideas, and many answers for yourself through the experiences and suggestions I share in *A Woman's Guide to Thriving after Prostate Cancer.*

Thank you for allowing me to share my discoveries so you can thrive, too.

With love, Cindie

Introduction

Women as Prostate Cancer Survivors

WHY THE TITLE *A Woman's Guide to Thriving after Prostate Cancer?* After all, women don't get prostate cancer. However, we hear about men getting this disease at an increasingly high rate. According to the American Cancer Society, there are more than two million men living in the United States who have been diagnosed with prostate cancer at some point in their life. That's a lot of men!

Because most men relate to more than one woman, the increasing number of men diagnosed with prostate cancer exponentially expands the number of women affected. Beyond being husbands or lovers, they connect to women as fathers, brothers, uncles, colleagues, and friends. Indeed, almost every woman I talk with shares a story about a man close to her who has (or has had) prostate cancer.

So how does this disease affect the women involved? In three ways: physically, emotionally, and spiritually.

Physical Impact

Most people think first about a woman's physical situation if she's in an intimate relationship with a man diagnosed with prostate cancer. I agree. Certainly, a woman's sex life can change significantly. Thus, much of this book provides ideas to help a woman look at sex in a whole new way. Chapter 2, Thriving Physically, provides tools to help her discover her unique definition of sexual fulfillment.

Even if your relationship with your man isn't sexual, this book provides two ways to help you thrive after prostate cancer: 1) You'll learn what your man's intimate partner may be experiencing and discover ways to support this person in her recovery, and 2) You'll gain ideas to improve your own sex life and otherwise enhance your happiness.

Admittedly, having sex with a partner changes after a prostate cancer diagnosis. I don't judge whether it's better or worse; it's just different. My experience proves that sex can become even more satisfying. As a bonus, what I learned isn't limited to couples recovering from prostate cancer. It can be valuable for anyone. If your sex life isn't thriving, read on. There's a lot here for you, especially in Chapter 2!

Emotional Impact

Prostate cancer can affect a woman emotionally in many ways. Whether your emotional pain came from hearing the dreaded words, "Your man has prostate cancer," from going through treatment with him, or from the devastation of your man dying, the ideas in this book will assist you.

Much of my prostate cancer experience hinged on the fear I felt, yet my fear diminished when I acquired knowledge. I learned to support my healing process with new communication skills, an understanding of my coping mechanisms, and the ability to look at my past differently.

When a friend recently described me as fearless, he didn't realize how much that meant to me. By releasing unhealthy emotional reactions to situations and becoming conscious of my true feelings, I now dwell in a fearless state most of the time. In Chapter 3, Thriving Emotionally, I share the techniques that freed me from my crippling fear.

Spiritual Impact

The third area in which a woman deals with prostate cancer involves her spirituality. In fact, any conversation about cancer invokes the thought of death and what happens after we leave our physical bodies. Once a woman hears a cancer diagnosis for a man she loves, she asks questions about his mortality. Soon after, she starts thinking about her own mortality—and maybe can't stop thinking about it for both of them.

In my situation, my heart closed down after Steve's diagnosis. I felt lost, disconnected from others, and especially disconnected from God. In many ways, I lived each day going through the motions, faking good feelings. I believed in the old adage "fake it till you make it."

Because Steve asked me to *not* share his diagnosis with others, I began to build a wall around me. I became more cautious about everything I said, wanting to make sure I honored his request. Although my wall started small, it grew bigger and stronger each day.

I found my heart diminishing, and I couldn't connect with others as easily as in the past. My heart, once relatively open, didn't feel free to love as before. So I lived the best way I knew how, smiling when I didn't feel happy, saying I felt fine when I didn't.

Looking back, I'm sure "faking it" helped in some ways. My spiritual life started to thrive, however, when I regained my sense of purpose—when I could foresee many gifts coming out of this prostate cancer experience. In effect, it began when I started asking for what I needed to experience those gifts. It continued as I tore down the wall I had built and started exploring my spirituality and relationship with my Higher Power.

It's Never Too Late

The most vital gift is knowing this: Whether your man had prostate cancer years ago or it has been recently diagnosed, it's never too late to learn *how* to thrive physically, emotionally, and spiritually. First and foremost, tap into the knowledge of other women; they can be your most powerful allies when it comes to turning surviving into thriving.

What is Thriving?

What do I mean by thriving? A woman who thrives after prostate cancer ideally lives a happy life, one that brings her fulfillment. She lives her passion by bringing her creative gifts into the world. She knows herself and how she can best serve others. She takes care of herself so she can take care of others.

For me, thriving means living the life of my dreams—that is, feeling sexually fulfilled, connected to my Higher Power, and aware of my feelings. My relationship with Steve feels blissful. I live in gratefulness for all the abundance in my life.

Thriving also means that I enjoy excellent health, I feel at peace, and my life flows effortlessly. I feel compassionate and serve others. I'm conscious of each moment, bringing love and laughter to each day. Instead of reacting to the situations that come my way, I consciously respond to them.

While I don't live a life that thrives like this every day, I keep my attention focused on these qualities. Every morning I set an intention to create a life that thrives. Because I know what I want, I'm able to create the life of my dreams more and more fully every day.

Create Your Vision of Thriving after Prostate Cancer

Right now, take a moment to contemplate and define what a thriving life looks like to you. By creating your unique definition, you become more focused on the life you want to enjoy now and in the future. Then ask your man to share his own definition.

Yes, you can gain the skills and find ways to thrive in all areas of your life. Remember, your life will "look" different after prostate cancer. Determine what a thriving life can look like for you. And don't try to fake it!

Ask So You Can Receive

Some of us try to do it all. Yet asking for assistance and learning to receive can help us thrive after prostate cancer. With an issue such as prostate cancer, women find it difficult to ask questions because many of them involve sex and sexuality—topics people often don't want to talk about or don't know how to answer pertinent questions.

Most people don't know what prostate cancer treatment does to a man's sexual function, plus each man responds differently to treatment. To make matters worse, a lack of knowledge exists about the prostate. Once, a male friend commented that many men don't even know where to find their prostate.

To get our questions answered about prostate cancer, most women seek private ways of obtaining information, searching websites and sometimes asking medical professionals to get clarity. In their book *Conscious Loving*, relationship experts Katie and Gay Hendricks recommend couples make statements in their communication, especially before asking a question.

Making a statement before asking a question can be as simple as saying to Steve, "I noticed you rubbing your scar from the prostate surgery. Would you like me to put lotion on the area for you?" If I didn't make a statement first, Steve might ask a clarifying question, or more likely, he would make an assumption about my intention. He might not be conscious of rubbing the area and ask me why I made the offer. Alternatively, he might assume that I wanted to be intimate together, potentially causing problems if all I wanted to do was eliminate his itching.

While it might sound like a simple thing to do, making statements doesn't come easily for me. Each time I do it, though, I find it so effective that I recommit myself to making more statements. I also find making statements—both at home and at work—helps me receive exactly the information I'm seeking.

Recently, I met with a man who I don't know very well to talk about a business matter. As we chatted before ordering lunch, he casually mentioned a recent medial experience. I asked if he wanted to share more, and he told me that his prostate had been removed three weeks ago.

He noted that many men at work didn't know much about the prostate gland and they asked him lots of questions. I let him know that Steve had been cancer-free for more than three years. I made a statement that I was writing this book and shared my desire to learn as much as I could from others.

Following that, I asked him, "What do you tell men about the prostate gland?" Because he knew why I asked, he gave me a very direct answer. He tells other men, "It's where the juice comes from." I found this information enlightening and appreciated his willingness to be so open with me, a relatively unknown business contact.

When I make a statement, I get the information I want, not what someone thinks I want. It allows the other person to let me know if he or she can't provide the information I seek. Plus it saves time and the potential embarrassment of the person not being able to help.

Draft Your Own Statements and Questions

You can help your recovery process by requesting that friends and family ask you questions about your prostate cancer experience. Make a statement first to let them know they can ask you anything. If you don't want to talk about a specific topic, like sex, make a statement that allows others to know you want to talk about your experience, except for your sex life.

Take some time to determine what you want to share with others. You might say something like, "I'm feeling great today because my husband celebrates three months of cancer-free living. I know we haven't talked much about this part of my life, and I'm ready to talk about anything except my sex life. That's still pretty private for me. Would you be willing to listen and ask questions about my prostate cancer experience?"

With others, you might consider a conversation like, "I'm feeling upset today. My brother called last night, and he's unhappy about his sex life after prostate cancer treatment. I'm glad he can talk with me about this topic, although I don't think I helped him much. Can we talk about ideas you have that will help me support him?"

Making statements like this encourages others to talk with you. If you don't open the door, they may avoid the subject of prostate cancer altogether. Also make a statement letting them know if you only want them to listen and not provide advice—something that's often more beneficial than getting advice.

Sometimes when I mention Steve's prostate treatment to people, they immediately change the subject. At first, I felt hurt and unhappy that they wouldn't talk with me. Now I believe the 'C' word, cancer, is probably frightening for them to discuss. They simply don't know what to say.

Some may have prostate cancer that hasn't been healed yet, or like Steve, they flat-out don't want to talk about it. Other times, people may know prostate cancer can affect a person's sexual function, and they don't want to talk about sex. I no longer take it personally when people don't want to talk about prostate cancer.

When I tell others about Steve's situation, I make sure to let them know right away that he is now in good health. Probably everyone we meet has experience with some type of cancer. Offering the reassuring news can quickly put the other person at ease.

It's best to talk about prostate cancer in our own ways. It's important to know our own boundaries and not allow others to cross them. When I keep my conversations technical and clinical, most people feel more at ease than when I speak about it from a personal perspective.

Each of us uses language differently. I can easily say the words "sex, ejaculation, and erection" but that's not true for Steve. He finds that using the word "intimacy" allows him to address the topic of sex in a more comfortable way.

I have found it helpful to tell people that sex is different after prostate cancer treatment, that the prostate gland secretes a liquid and without a healthy prostate, a man can't ejaculate, or he ejaculates just a small amount. It doesn't mean he can't have orgasms, and it doesn't mean he can't obtain an erection. It simply means the physical act of ejaculating a fluid doesn't happen anymore.

Regular prostate exams and living a healthy lifestyle can reduce risks of prostate cancer. Many people don't know that a man can consider many different treatments if his prostate becomes unhealthy. I make sure people know it's especially important for a man to receive treatment, if recommended, to help him stay healthy.

By holding these educational conversations, I hope to prevent misconceptions. A friend told me about a man who believed so strongly that he couldn't experience satisfying sex after treatment for prostate cancer that he didn't get treatment. He died from the cancer a few years later. This doesn't need to happen!

Staying Present—Because It Works

Steve and I had been through so much—his enlarged prostate, the cancer diagnosis, his surgery and recovery. To add to our stress, during this same period, the man my mom had been married to for 20 years passed away. Then, a year after Steve's diagnosis, my mom was diagnosed with early Alzheimer's disease. Her care fell to me and to my sister. (She lives across the country while I live two hours away.) Steve and I found ourselves faced with many unfamiliar situations during two of the darkest years of our lives. Writing that sentence still brings up a lot of emotion remembering the pain I felt during that time.

Cry, Sob, Dance, Run

Do you have similar feelings as you recall your situation during your prostate cancer experience? If so, I invite you to do what I just did. I found a quiet place and cried, and cried, and cried some more. I breathed deeply and let out lots of sounds.

Then I moved my body. I felt a lot of tension in my hips and lower back area, so I practiced my belly dancing-like jiggles, moving all the energy out that I brought up by going back to that time of pain.

Cry, sob, dance, run, or do something physical. It helps you eliminate any unhealthy emotions your body still holds as you continue to experience that time in your life or recall it. No matter what else life brings you at the time of the prostate cancer diagnosis, your emotional state is strongly affected.

Right before Steve's surgery, a friend mentioned climbing Camelback Mountain. It had been more than five years since I'd hiked that beautiful trail in the middle of Phoenix. I decided to get away from it all, spend time alone getting exercise, and contemplate my life while I hiked.

Hiking Camelback Mountain brought me peace. In fact, I found hiking—or walking in my neighborhood if I didn't want to take time to hike—brought me into a healing space like no other activity. That alone time in nature gave me just what I required to clear my head, contemplate Steve's diagnosis, and regain some semblance of normalcy. That feeling of normalcy helped me stay centered as events swirled around me.

Because I hiked early in the morning, I didn't see many people, allowing me to feel more of my emotions and breathe more deeply as I walked. Listening to the birds, observing the cactuses, and feeling the air temperature on my skin, I focused hard to stay present. Anything to keep my mind off of "real life." Anything to provide me relief from a relationship with Steve that didn't work well at the time. Anything to postpone grieving the loss of the mother I knew.

My mind tugged at me to go forward in time, to worry about the future. Or it dragged me into the past to ruminate about things I'd said or not said—often something that didn't even matter, yet I couldn't let it go.

My mom's illness, more than Steve's, taught me about staying present—or not. I found myself going into the future, wondering how we'd find the money for her care, wondering how much of my time her care would take, wondering what hereditary health issues my sister and I might face, and on and on. So many possibilities! My imagination worked overtime.

As I kept searching for answers and exploring different techniques, I discovered that when I stayed present, my energy increased and I could really enjoy that moment. Reading Pema Chödrön's book *When Things Fall Apart* provided me with new insights. When I lived one moment at a time, I gained strength to handle whatever came my way. My energy became more focused and abundant because I didn't spend it in unproductive ways.

As I learned these new techniques around my mom's situation, I started transferring them to my relationship with

Steve. Staying present gave me more energy to devote to our relationship. Yet I could still easily slip back to the past—to times of pre-prostate problems. Sometimes I liked wallowing in self-pity and complaining to others about the unfortunate hand I'd been dealt.

Specifically, I found it much easier to complain about Steve's emotional unavailability and our lack of closeness than to take responsibility for my part in the situation. In reality, that didn't make it easier, and it kept me locked in the past, not moving forward.

Yet, when I stayed focused in the present and just lived in each moment, I found I didn't complain as much. I also didn't ask those questions: What if Steve hadn't gotten prostate cancer? What if my mom could take care of herself? What if my sex life were as great as it was years ago?

Living in the present moment allows me to stay conscious, aware of my surroundings, my feelings, and my health. I'm more capable of making wise decisions in this space than in other spaces. I'm more able to keep my emotions from taking over my life and to *respond* instead of *react* to situations that upset me.

Along the way, a colleague introduced me to Faye Mandell whose book *Self-Powerment* provided additional techniques to help me live in the now. This small book of only 176 pages gave me many practical ways to stay present.

In particular, the author shared a methodology I use when my mind escapes into the past or future. She included a chart that makes it easy to figure out where I am when I'm not present and to quickly work through an issue to get back to the moment.

A year ago, I found myself worrying about Steve's health and reliving his prostate surgery. Steve came home from working out at the gym, noting that a funny bump had appeared in his groin area. Sure enough, after seeing a doctor, he received a hernia diagnosis.

This situation brought up the same thoughts and emotions for me that arose when he received his prostate cancer diagnosis. I wondered whether he would be around in the future and what life would look like without him.

Sitting in the hospital waiting room during Steve's hernia surgery, I relived the terror I felt seeing him in the pre-op room. You know—that helpless feeling seeing my man hooked up with tubes, wearing that hospital gown, right before he goes under the anesthesia. As I waited for Steve, my thoughts flew into the future, wondering what else might happen to his health.

Using the techniques in Faye Mandell's book, I discovered that when my thoughts were pulled back to the past, I typically wasn't feeling adequate. Indeed, I was experiencing guilt about a situation at a time when I needed to feel sadness and disappointment about what had happened. Plus I still needed to grieve around the issue of Steve's health and accept the fact that I did the best I could back when he received his diagnosis.

My thoughts about the future typically related to feeling afraid. Since then, I've found ways to reduce or eliminate my fear by gaining knowledge. I ask more questions and spend more time on research when I find myself worrying about a future event. These techniques and resources, in addition to those already noted, provide me with ways to stay present. When I don't allow myself to go into the past or the future—when I take life just one moment at a time—everything becomes much easier for me.

I still plan ahead to make sure my mom receives the care she requires; I schedule intimacy sessions with Steve on my calendar; I continue to celebrate experiences in the past. But I find that life flows much more easily when I live right now—in the present moment.

We're Prostate Cancer Survivors, Too!

Many books and medical professionals don't view women as prostate cancer survivors. I strongly disagree. I believe a woman who supports a man through his prostate cancer diagnosis and treatment can proudly wear the title of prostate cancer survivor.

Without doubt, women affected by prostate cancer want to help their man heal, to "fix" him and make him "all better." They want their man to regain his health and live cancer-free. Women traditionally play the role of caretaker, wanting family and friends to live happy, healthy lives.

Yet many women don't realize this critical factor: *To help her man get better and live a healthy life, the woman must heal herself first.* Yes, healing ourselves comes FIRST!

Often, as women, we don't like to hear this. We want to tap into our innate urge to turn our attention to our man, nurturing him through his recovery process. Not surprisingly, we tend to ignore our own needs because we're focused on our man and the rest of the family. We may view our own success based on the apparent success of those around us. Thus, we view our man's recovery as our own recovery.

In the beginning, I've learned, this is an essential approach. Adept at multitasking, we mobilize our lives to reprioritize our activities and help him decide what treatment to choose. Not only do we support our man during his treatment, he needs our support while he's regaining his health after treatment. Oh, how we love to celebrate the news of his first zero PSA test result!

At some point, though, our man moves out of the danger zone. That's when I suggest migrating the attention to our own recovery process—which is unwise to neglect, ignore, or postpone. Ever!

Yet, too often, we don't do this. Instead, we continue focusing on our man, helping him regain his life after prostate cancer. By doing so, we ignore one of the most important parts of *his* healing process: *our own healing.* We often hear, "If Mama ain't happy, no one is happy." This suggests the value of women living a happy life after prostate cancer.

This guide focuses on how *you* as a woman can learn to thrive after prostate cancer, not on how you can help your man thrive—although that could well be a by-product of focusing on your own wellness.

Your man's recovery process may look similar to yours or it may be extremely different. What you learn about your own healing, though, will provide you with many tools that can assist your man with his recovery. *He* gains the opportunity to thrive because *you* live a life that's magnificent!

CHAPTER 1

GRIEVING THE LOSSES

WHEN I HEARD STEVE say those dreaded words, "I have prostate cancer," I didn't realize how much cold water this would throw on my life. Knowing the diagnosis related to *his* body, I assumed the recovery process would be all about *him*. Yet, when my own feelings of happiness didn't return after his treatment, I realized the tremendous impact his diagnosis had on me.

Once I saw that I required healing from prostate cancer too, it took me a while to accept that my own healing needed to be an inside job. Before then, I had looked outside myself for answers. I believed Steve needed to change; I thought our relationship needed an overhaul; I searched for dozens of possibilities.

My "Ah Ha" Moment

My "ah ha" moment occurred in June 2008. I traveled to San Francisco to take a class called Celebrating Women: Regarding Ecstasy and Power™, one year after Steve and I visited a doctor at the University of San Francisco Medical Center to obtain another opinion on his diagnosis and explore treatment options.

There, I learned to become a "Queen" with more than 75 other women. I kept my attention focused on me. I set an intention to learn about my requirements and desires, then to learn how to fulfill them. I also intended to discover new ways to express my creativity, my femininity, and my sexuality.

Through lectures, conversations, exercises, journaling, and speaking, I learned the importance of taking care of myself, how to give, and how to receive. I discovered the qualities I want to embody. I decided to *become* a Queen. I understood the benefits to me, to Steve, and to our relationship.

I committed to learn how to be happy and fulfilled, allowing me to bring energy and life to those around me. I vowed to look inside, as frightening as that felt, and to heal anything that got in the way.

I began to understand that no one could do the work for me—that Steve didn't have the power to make me happy. I also realized I didn't possess all the skills needed to completely recover; I needed others to assist me. So I asked for support and found it in many places.

At the end of her *O* magazine, Oprah writes on the topic of "What I Know for Sure." It got me to ask myself that question. What I know for sure is this: *The only way for me to thrive after prostate cancer is to heal myself.* Healing meant looking at my life and my way of responding to situations. Most profoundly, it required me to get to know myself.

I also had to accept that my own recovery didn't depend on Steve's recovery. I couldn't judge my recovery by Steve's progress; his healing and his recovery remained with him, not with me. Nor could I take responsibility for Steve's recovery (as I had tried to do at first). My mantra became I'm not responsible for his recovery. I can't change him. I can only change myself.

The lessons learned have been painful and difficult—and highly necessary. Among the most important is realizing that, as women, we can assist each other to heal. As we do, we give increasingly more compassion to ourselves. And because of that, we can provide more compassion to the men in our lives.

Why Grief Has to Be Part of the Equation

It takes exploring the pain and grief that surface as part of this diagnosis. Yes, I include grief in this equation because to survive any immense change means to experience loss. And loss goes hand in hand with grief.

I didn't read much about grieving during or after my experience with prostate cancer. After all, Steve has been able to live a healthy life after his treatment. He didn't die, so why would grieving apply to me?

My answer came one year after Steve's diagnosis. After reading the book *The 36-Hour Day*, I went back to the following passage, "We usually think of grief as an emotional experience that follows a death. However, grief is a natural emotional response to loss . . . ." This book (actually a guide for families caring for those with Alzheimer's disease) held the key for me to heal!

Then, I suddenly realized that I hadn't fully immersed myself into the grieving process after all the losses I experienced as a result of prostate cancer. Today, I realize that any time I lose something—when life changes in some way big or small—I must grieve. Change never ceases. I might have to cancel a vacation or forfeit a lunch with friends because something changed. Addressing events like these involves two steps: 1) feeling the pain of loss in my body, and 2) allowing myself time to heal that pain.

Even if the loss leads to a desired improvement—like getting a promotion at work—I'm still leaving behind things I value, such as the camaraderie of my former co-workers. What I've learned is paramount: *I have to grieve that loss so I can move forward.* In fact, I've learned that going through a *healthy* grieving process can move me from surviving to thriving in a short time—and it can for you, too.

5 Stages of Grief

Once a woman hears that prostate cancer diagnosis as I did, she grieves a number of losses, although each person grieves differently. Those who counsel in this area provide commonly accepted steps to help people get through any loss—the five stages of grief are: denial, anger, bargaining, depression, and acceptance.

These stages of grief were first introduced by Elisabeth Kübler-Ross in her book *On Death and Dying.* Kübler-Ross didn't believe that all steps are experienced after each loss and noted that the steps don't necessarily come in the order stated here. While some find a natural resilience to be a common response to loss, I appreciate the formulaic approach of understanding loss through these five stages.

I also understand that each time I grieve a loss, my experience will be unique. I may spend a differing amount of time in each stage depending on the significance of the loss; I may not experience one or more of the stages; I may easily recover from a loss. After reaching the acceptance stage, I periodically bounce back into other stages, but eventually, I live in the acceptance stage most of the time.

Often people don't understand the need for another person to go through the grieving process. They don't know how to support them even though they want to. Listeners who have the best intentions find it uncomfortable to hear how someone feels at a deep level. And when someone talks about his or her loss, it reminds listeners of the losses and pains from their own lives that they've buried and ignored.

When I grieve a loss, I remind myself of the five stages (sometimes referred to as phases). I figure out where I am in the process, allowing myself time in each stage that's needed and time to bounce back and forth between stages. When talking with someone who's experienced a loss, understanding these five stages allows me to assist that person through the stage of grief he or she is experiencing.

Through a series of questions and active listening, we can determine which of the five stages a person is in. Once we know this, we can support the person appropriately and possibly suggest that they seek professional counseling. If someone denies a loss, we can gently provide facts that can help the person move forward.

When someone expresses anger, we can match their emotion for a time, supporting them in releasing these feelings in a healthy way. During the bargaining stage, we can listen, help them become aware of their behavior, and provide suggestions for resolution.

Unfortunately, most people in our culture don't deal well with the fourth stage, depression. Too many people tell others to "Just get over it" or "It's time to move on" before the person is ready to move into the fifth stage—acceptance. Naturally, we don't like seeing others in pain; we want them to "get better" right away. "Life goes on," we declare. Yet, we're actually dismissing what's really going on—and missing a golden opportunity to heal.

To Those Who Are Grieving

What can we offer those who are grieving? A listening ear and a genuine concern for how they feel. It's rare that retelling our own experiences brings them comfort. Words about us can seem hollow and meaningless to the person in pain. Simply offering to listen to *their* stories and feelings, hugging them, and saying "Tell me more" can bring solace to a grieving person.

As I write this, four years after Steve's diagnosis, I still grieve. I haven't fully accepted the necessary changes. And I'm okay with that. The good news? These days, I find myself moving quickly through the stages, frequently skipping the denial and bargaining stages. Anger and depression still haunt me on occasion, but most of the time, I live in the realm of acceptance. "What is" is okay with me.

The Grieving Process

Once I understood more about the grieving process, I realized I'd lost a great deal before Steve even got his diagnosis. For years, Steve lived with an enlarged prostate and received regular biopsies. Knowing the painful biopsies weren't pleasant, we were both concerned. As a result, we didn't have much of a sex life, losing the intimacy we'd enjoyed years before.

Like many men who eventually receive a prostate cancer diagnosis, Steve's enlarged prostate affected his ability to achieve an erection. Admittedly, we didn't do a good job of finding alternatives to sexual intercourse. Instead, we ignored the problem. Our relationship suffered. We got used to not having sex, which affected our bonding as a couple. For three years, we benignly lived with this big elephant in the room. Still, at the time, I didn't view this as a loss that I needed to grieve. I do now.

Then came the words, "Your husband has prostate cancer." The meaning behind those words took away my dreams and the future I'd envisioned. Specifically, Steve and I were creating a business around a book I had written to help people reduce the hassles in their lives. My vision of a life working with my husband, assisting other people in a meaningful way, went down the drain with the "C" word. People can change dramatically from cancer treatment and some lose their lives to the disease. I didn't know what life would look like next month, much less next year.

The diagnosis also caused me to lose communication with my husband. As soon as Steve heard those words himself, he retreated inwardly. At that point, I lost the little intimacy we had retained. I lost my sense of being desired and being attractive to the man I loved. I lost my sense of security that Steve would be around for a long time—and we were losing our valuable time together. I knew that couples could lose their marriages if they couldn't repair their relationships after prostate treatment. I was also acutely aware that some women suffer the ultimate loss—their man dies.

Although I felt immense loss at the time of Steve's diagnosis, how could I take a moment to grieve when we needed to focus on Steve's survival? Wasn't it my job, as his wife, to help him make it through his treatment regimen?

Yes, absolutely.

So, my grieving process would have to wait. And your grieving likely had to wait, too.

Sure, I grieved some in the form of my anger often surfacing and feeling sad, even depressed, following his diagnosis. Regardless of any reaction, though, we had to face facts. Steve had cancer. So we soldiered on, focusing fully on his treatment path.

Whatever Stage You're in Now, Write Down Your Losses

Did you make your man's health a priority, too? I hope he's recovered and I also hope he took time to grieve. I know Steve and I didn't grieve soon enough or long enough. Why? Because I didn't realize the importance of going through the grieving process, especially for me—and if you're on a similar path, it's the same for you, too.

Create your own list of losses you've experienced due to prostate cancer. Remember, you can only fully grieve your losses when you become aware of them.

Grieving the Physical Losses

Denial: When I consciously started grieving, I could see how I denied the loss of our physical relationship. I convinced myself that our life wasn't so bad after all, and that sex wasn't that important to our relationship. I denied I felt unhappy about the shrinking of our intimate relationship. I rationalized that I would "make do" with holding hands and sleeping next to each other.

Anger: I looked back and saw my anger about the loss of our sex life. I felt anger at Steve for not initiating sex. I felt anger when he had difficulty getting an erection. I didn't blame him. I understood the health issue. Yet I still felt angry when I couldn't feel him inside me.

Bargaining: Then I bargained with Steve as we searched for ways to improve our sex life. We came up with agreements to make having sex amenable for both of us.

Depression: The depression stage stayed with me the longest. I felt a lot of sadness both before and after his diagnosis. I didn't feel any passion for our physical relationship or for my life in general. Deep down, I just felt undesired and unloved.

Grieving the Emotional Losses

Denial: For a time, I denied the fact that we lost our emotional connection, or perhaps I just didn't want to admit it. I kept thinking his response to the diagnosis was probably normal, and that all would be okay once he'd decided on a treatment. But when our emotional connection didn't get better, I went into denial again. Everything would be fine after his surgery, I told myself.

Anger: I felt a lot of anger about losing Steve emotionally. After the diagnosis, he retreated into himself, and I couldn't find a way to reach him. Unable to talk with him, I didn't know how he felt. Because Steve didn't know how he felt either, he couldn't verbalize what was going on for him. It seemed like he went into survival mode and could only give attention to his own experience. He couldn't talk with me about my feelings at all. Everything revolved around him. Not surprisingly, I felt abandoned, alone.

Bargaining: I certainly bargained with Steve emotionally. I attempted to talk to him and asked a lot of questions that he couldn't answer. I suggested he talk with a counselor to assist him. But he attended just one appointment and only because I scheduled it for him.

Depression: I spun into a form of depression when I couldn't get answers from Steve. Because he barely talked to me after his diagnosis and before his surgery, I moved into something that felt like a black hole. I still felt all alone.

Grieving the Spiritual Losses

Denial: I don't know why I didn't turn to God during this time of pain. Often when we can't talk to others about our feelings and troubles, we turn to God. I didn't. Most likely my relationship with my Higher Power wasn't strong enough at the time. It felt more comfortable to take my usual independent approach and "do it myself," denying myself this opportunity to deepen my spirituality.

Anger: I didn't know why this had happened to me. I was angry, questioning my spiritual beliefs and wondering why prostate cancer struck us. I felt that God had abandoned us—that if He really loved us, He wouldn't have allowed my man to get prostate cancer. I was angry at God, doubting His existence.

Bargaining: I don't remember bargaining with God, most likely because my heart was closed and I felt very alone. I believe it's pretty common to bargain with God in this circumstance, though. Perhaps you remember offering God a deal, praying that He make your man cancer-free in exchange for you becoming a better wife, mother, or daughter. You may remember committing to attend church once a week, vowing to read the Bible every day, or promising to never ask for anything again—only if God would help your man get rid of the cancer.

Depression: During the long months I hung out in this stage, I felt lethargic. I found myself avoiding Steve. I drank more alcohol than usual; I went hiking a lot; I worked long hours. I did anything to escape my fear that Steve might die and that our marriage was crumbling. I didn't want to lose him. I didn't want my third marriage to end in divorce.

My faith in God, my connection with my Higher Power, diminished, causing me to remain depressed. Did I say I felt alone?

Periodically, I remembered the beautiful story of Jesus walking next to someone on a sandy beach—the picture of two pairs of footprints in the sand side by side, then suddenly, just one set. Most of this time, I believed that Jesus deserted me during my time of need and that I was walking on the beach alone.

Deep down, though, I knew that Jesus didn't leave me during that difficult time. Instead, I knew He carried me when I was too weak to walk, leaving His one set of footprints, not mine. A few times, I could believe Jesus carried me.

Remembering I wasn't alone—and knowing that assistance came from something bigger than me—brought me comfort. Sometimes. Yet during my darkest days, nothing seemed to comfort me.

Music and Grieving

For two years after Steve's diagnosis, I denied myself the opportunity to use this grieving process to dig deep into the feelings beneath my pain. I didn't want to bring those memories forward again. It hurt too much.

But eventually, I realized that I had to take the time—to find the courage—to process all my grief so I could experience true healing. If my wounds remained covered yet unhealed, they were in danger of infection. I decided to use music to process my stages of grief. So in my anger stage, I played protest music—loudly—so I could let out those raw, angry emotions. The Dixie Chicks's album *Taking the Long Way* became my anthem. Their angry statements of purpose and resolve, coupled with vulnerability and defiance, spoke to me. The raw emotions in the songs motivated me to dance, moving energy stuck in my body. It made me feel powerful and alive, qualities I hadn't felt for quite some time.

Sometimes, I chose music to accompany my depression. While I didn't create a playlist of gloomy blues tunes, I played a handful of songs over and over again to match my mood. One dark night, I blasted Paul Davis's tune "I Go Crazy" through my headphones for about an hour without a break.

Once, while I was out of town at a board meeting for a nonprofit organization, I drank too much wine at dinner and couldn't sleep. I decided to mourn the hand life had dealt me. Memories came flooding through my body of all the magical sexual experiences I had enjoyed in that town with a special man from my youth. That's when I deeply grieved the loss of my sex life with Steve, tears pouring down my cheeks.

In my version of going crazy, I danced to this song while emitting painful, silent cries from my throat. Exhausted, I finally fell asleep around 3 a.m., rising three hours later to go for a walk with a good friend. I kept my sunglasses on so he wouldn't notice my swollen eyes. I'm sure he wondered why my voice was so hoarse.

While I physically felt rotten that morning, I made it through the board meeting, drove home, and got a good night's sleep. The next day, I felt at peace, more open and clear. Still emotional, I felt unsure about what had happened and what to do next.

Create Your Own Grieving Music

Develop a musical playlist for all, or some, of the five stages of grief. Crank up the volume on your selected favorites to move energy through and out of your body. Use it to cry your deepest tears and release them to the universe.

Ahhh—Acceptance, Finally

I wish I could say I came across one marvelous, surefire way to grieve all my losses. I can't. Instead, my path to thriving came from the combination of traditional and nontraditional healing methods that I explain throughout this book. At this writing, I'm on my way to feeling close to 95 percent healed.

Today, I still work many more than 40 hours each week at a job I love. I hike Camelback Mountain two to three times a week. And I enjoy weekly intimate time with Steve. I don't numb myself with alcohol any more. Most of the time, I consciously respond to situations rather than react to them based on triggers from my past. Finally, my life thrives!

When pain arises, and it still does, I breathe into it and experience my feelings, no matter how much they hurt. Writing this book brought up emotions I thought (and hoped) had disappeared. They hadn't. I cried a zillion tears as I re-experienced the fear and the pain of those years when "just existing" as a prostate cancer survivor numbed my senses.

What I Learned About Men

During my prostate cancer experience, I learned a lot about men. I realized that most men respond to survival situations differently than women. Specifically, men take care of themselves first so they can take care of their partners later. While I thought Steve was acting selfishly by not attending to my needs, I now know he simply *couldn't* respond to my needs. He had to focus on himself to eliminate the cancer from his body.

At the time, I didn't realize his way of showing his love for me meant making his own health a priority. After all, if he didn't get healthy, he couldn't take care of me in the future. Today, I accept that many men don't verbalize their feelings well. While I resist acknowledging that fact, I now better understand how men and women differ in this area. These days, I ask Steve more questions than I ever did, and then I wait. Usually, I feel okay when he can't give me an answer.

My process also involved grieving my idealized version of my marriage. I wanted Steve to respond to situations in ways similar to how I'd normally respond. But he can't. I now realize that. And today, much more than ever, I value the differences between the two of us and strive to consciously build on each of our strengths.

Own Your Own Grieving Journey

On your own journey to recovery, please grieve and grieve thoroughly. Experience each of the five stages of grieving for *all* your losses—whether they're from prostate cancer or other situations. Know that the rewards are imminent. Believe that you will live in the acceptance stage and fully appreciate your life for the treasure it is. Then you can truly thrive after prostate cancer.

CHAPTER 2

THRIVING PHYSICALLY

LOOKING BACK, I can clearly see that I didn't address the physical changes related to Steve's prostate cancer soon enough. Not just the physical changes after his treatment but those that occurred before his diagnosis.

I saw signs of trouble but ignored them. Steve's enlarged prostate made it difficult for him to achieve an erection. Perhaps I subconsciously rationalized it away as a cooling of passion that often happens to couples over the years when other demands of life abound.

Also, I admit I didn't *want* to spend time on our sex life, so I distracted myself with numerous other activities. I was avoiding sex to escape the fear of intimacy that arose in me when I would get too close to Steve—despite the enjoyable and blissful feelings I could create during our times of closeness.

Facing Fears Around Sex
Complete intimacy still eludes me at times because of my fears, but less frequently than before I realized (during the "Queen"

course) that feeling happy and fulfilled is an inside job. As I continue to learn how to surrender into intimacy and feel safe in that space, my joy increases and my own health improves.

Yes, scientific and medical studies have proven repeatedly that sex is good for one's health. Women who enjoy a fulfilling sex life probably already realize that sex helps them look and feel younger. And who doesn't want that? So why don't the rest of us spend more time with sex? Why do we allow ourselves to be drawn in other directions and avoid this special time with our man? Most often, it's because we're afraid . . . but of what?

Great intimate relationships that include mind-blowing sexual activity require us to be vulnerable. With our feelings exposed, unknown fears or those related to past events arise.

Everyone holds different beliefs about sex and has varying experiences around it, but one thing is common: We don't talk about sex easily. Our society doesn't encourage conversations about this topic, so we hide our beliefs, feelings, and experiences. We stuff them away. Thus we don't know if our experiences are "normal," which may cause us even more anxiety.

Because we don't often compare our experiences with others, we also don't create as many opportunities to learn about sex as we could. We converse effortlessly for hours on topics like cooking, travel, and parenting. Only in special relationships do we allow ourselves the opportunity to share stories about our sex life and ask questions of others.

In addition, many women have experienced traumatic sexual events as children, adults, or both. No matter when our trauma occurred or how often, most of us carry a lot of baggage when it comes to sex.

Staying Present

Your interest in this book indicates your readiness to change your life or help someone you know change hers. Of course, you want to help your man thrive after his brush with death, but you also want your own life to improve. You may have tried many things but haven't quite found the key.

As a woman who has found and uses a lot of keys, I summarize the best way to thrive physically after prostate cancer with these two magic words: *Stay present.* Similar phrases might be: *Live in the now, Be here right now, Be in the moment.* However, although these words are simple to write and easy to say, they are innately difficult to achieve. Is that true for you, too?

Yet I still believe strongly in this key. Why? Because it works! Having assimilated many books, programs, conferences, and other experiences, I know for sure that staying present changes my life for the better in every way. It simply works better than anything else I've learned.

Staying in the present moment during sex especially keeps my attention focused *in the now* where safety exists. My mind doesn't wander to past upsetting experiences, and it doesn't drag me forward to what might happen in the future. I feel safe in the now.

Creating a Safe Space

What is a safe space? To me, it's a place that's free from intruders and distractions, and an environment where emotional security can be achieved. While this may seem basic, I find that many women haven't considered what safety means to them. So first let's discuss creating a safe physical space to help us stay present during sex. Then let's determine how to feel emotionally secure.

Physical Safety

What does safety mean to you? Safety may mean time alone with the doors locked, with everyone out of the house, including your man. Yes, we can enjoy sex alone, and often this time alone provides an opportunity to get to know our sexual selves better.

Creating a safe space may mean talking with your man about your fears, opening up to get his attention and his support. Few men understand the world women live in with respect to our concern for our physical safety. One of the most powerful examples of getting a man's attention in this area is an exercise I've participated in during several different training programs. Let me explain.

During class, the men and women divide into different groups and list all the things they do to keep themselves physically safe. The men stand around for a while and finally write a few words on their flip chart page. During this time, they shake their heads in amazement as they glance over at the women who are actively writing words on their flip chart pages. When the exercise ends, the men look in astonishment at the *four pages* of items created by the women compared to their half-page.

As the facilitator debriefs the exercise, men realize that women constantly monitor the environment to make sure we remain physically safe. They look surprised when we show them how we hold our keys when walking to our cars. They didn't realize that we look behind the shower curtain in a hotel and under the bed any time we return to our room. They're surprised to learn how we survey parking lots and move our car closer to the office door when planning to work late.

What You Do to Stay Physically Safe

Make a list of the habits you've acquired to help you stay safe. Consider brainstorming with girlfriends to discover items you forgot or to gather new ideas. Ask yourself when you were last afraid for your physical safety, then ask your man. Most likely, you'll find two very different answers. Then share your list with him, allowing him to experience your world.

I believe most men want to support us but often don't know how, *and* we don't know how to ask for their support. Having a conversation with your man in this way will get his attention and support.

Men pride themselves in their ability to protect their women. However, we often don't allow them to do so, or don't share with them what we require to feel safe. I didn't do this well for many years. I expected Steve to read my mind and know what I required. I didn't know that a big part of what I required to enjoy sex related to safety and feeling protected. Steve could easily provide this for me if he knew I wanted a secure environment.

Mostly, I didn't want to admit my weakness and fear. I'm an independent woman. I can take care of myself, or so I thought. I didn't realize the dynamics between a healthy couple—the importance of assigning roles to each other and supporting each other in those roles. I thought I needed to "do it all"—and did a good job of it.

However, over the years, I learned it didn't help my marriage to "do it all." Not only did it prevent Steve from contributing to our relationship, it didn't allow me to take a break and relax. I was constantly on guard, protecting all the time.

Steve used to travel quite a bit, so I made sure I stayed safe while I was home alone. When he returned, I continued to take that responsibility, not realizing that was something he wanted to do and could do easily. In truth, my need to control, to be in charge, exhausted me. Plus it didn't allow Steve to provide an important role at home and in our marriage.

I began using the word *surrender* to assist me in overcoming my need to control and stay in charge. When I truly embodied the concept of surrender, it allowed me to look at my life with Steve completely differently. I could relax and stay present with him, allowing him to provide a safety net for me from the world.

Even though we live in a relatively crime-free area and implement precautions against intruders, I still have concerns for the safety of my body. That just seems to be the world I live in. Fear doesn't dominate my life. I simply want to be aware and smart when it comes to my physical safety.

As I learned to surrender control, I discovered that Steve could make sure my physical body remained safe and that our intimate times together were free from distractions. If I felt physically protected and knew I wouldn't be disturbed, I could stay in the present moment more easily. That meant I could enjoy sex more.

I admit, in the past, I didn't communicate my needs to Steve very well. By reading about communication between couples, taking classes to learn about what men prefer, and gaining skills to provide feedback at work, I found an effective way to ask for assistance. Here's how it works: I first need to get Steve's attention and let him know I have something important to say. We schedule a time to talk. My goal? To market my idea to him in such a way that he will be interested in talking with me in depth. I then tell him, in as few words as possible, what I want and ask if he's willing to help. If he is, we specifically review the information and I obtain his agreement on the final action(s). Then I ask if there's anything I can do to support him. At the end, I thank him and express how I feel because of his assistance.

A Communication Style That Works Well

See if the following dialogue helps you let your man know what he can do to make sure you feel safe and obtain his commitment to provide it for you. I resisted this type of communication style until I found out *it works every time.*

"Steve, may I interrupt you for just a minute? I want to arrange a time to share something important. I never asked you to help me feel safe in specific ways. When would be a good time to talk about this?"

"How about after lunch? Is that soon enough?"

"Yes, thank you."

"It's after lunch, Steve. Thanks for taking time to talk. I learned something about myself and our sex life today. I discovered that I can enjoy sex more if I feel safe. I think you can help me feel safe in several ways. Would you be willing to do that?"

"Tell me what you want."

"Feeling physically safe helps me relax. Can you make sure our home is secure and protected from intruders before our intimate times together?"

"I can do that. I'll make sure the doors are locked. Do you want me to turn on the house alarm?"

"No. That's not necessary."

"What else can I do?"

"Please make sure the phone won't ring. I'll turn off my cell phone. It will help if you turn off your cell phone and unplug the land line."

"Okay, I can do that. Anything else, Cindie?"

"Just one more thing, Steve. Please share with me your understanding of what you'll do to help me feel safe."

"You want me to secure the house so you feel physically safe before our intimacy sessions. I'll do that by locking the doors and making sure the phones don't ring. Is that right?"

"Yes. Steve, are you willing to do that to help me?"

"Yes."

"How can I support you in doing this for me?"

"Don't get mad at me if I forget. You can remind me to make sure the doors are locked and the phones are turned off."

"I can do that. By doing this for me, Steve, you'll allow me to relax and be more present during our intimacy sessions. That way I can enjoy our special time together more. Thank you for making sure I feel safe."

When I first started communicating with Steve in this way, it felt odd. I didn't feel comfortable talking in short sentences, asking him to repeat his understanding of our conversation and clearly stating my request. It felt different to let him know what his actions would provide for me.

Communicating like this also took me more time to prepare, something I didn't want to do. In the long run, however, I found the investment of time well worth the effort. I often wasn't clear on what I wanted and that confused Steve, causing him to tune out rather than listen to me and meet my needs.

Through just this one conversation, Steve's agreeing to help me feel safe allowed me to stay in the present moment with him during sex. As I started using this communication model, I found Steve being more aware of meeting my needs in multiple areas of our lives.

Emotional Safety

Creating a safe space includes feeling safe emotionally with Steve. I didn't quite know what that meant, so I had to figure it out. And guess what? I discovered that safety—like so many other things—is an inside job. I just hadn't realized this before.

A year ago, I joined an organization that assists CEOs become better leaders. During my initial meeting with my group leader, he asked me what it would take to feel safe with the others CEOs in the group, thus creating a trusting relationship. An answer came to me immediately, and since it sounded too simple, I kept searching for a more profound response.

Since one didn't come, I shared that there wasn't anything the other CEOs could do to help me feel safe. It was up to me! With respect to trust, I concluded that I would trust the other members of the group until a behavior showed me that a CEO didn't warrant my trust. This discovery fit with my earlier conclusion that my happiness and fulfillment is an inside job. I was able to answer my group leader's question about the CEO group in this way because, at this point in my business career, I feel safe in most situations.

Not so in my relationship with Steve, I realized. Remember that chant from grade school "stick and stones may break my bones, but names will never harm me"? That's what I'm talking about. Steve can help me feel safe with his actions, but bottom line, I must give emotional safety to myself.

What does this feeling of emotional safety involve? It means trusting myself and knowing who I am. It means living authentically, feeling centered, and loving myself. If I feel used or if my feelings get hurt, it's my cue to go inside and understand what baggage from the past is causing those emotions.

As much as I didn't want to accept this fact, I finally realized that *Steve doesn't make me feel a specific way.* It's much easier to look for excuses on the outside, putting the blame on someone or something else. I had grown up in that kind of environment, as most people do.

Through my quest for increased self-awareness, I put the pieces together from the books I read, classes I attended, and counseling I received. Just like when my inner voice answered the question from my CEO group leader so quickly, eventually my inner voice came through and confirmed that my emotional safety could only come from within me.

Making a shift in my way of thinking would take courage. And a lot of it. I knew Steve's actions could trigger certain reactions within me. If I react in an unhealthy way, it's my job to determine what caused this response and then learn how to respond in a healthy way. In the past, it was much easier to hold him responsible or criticize him for doing something wrong.

Once I knew what safety meant to me, I explored ways I could create it in my life, which I describe in Chapter 3, Thriving Emotionally. Ensuring feelings of safety became a giant step toward thriving after prostate cancer.

Breathing and Making Sounds

Once you begin to feel safe, we can explore ways to stay in the present moment. One technique that sounds simple yet may not be easy is deep breathing—in my view, the best way to become present in an instant.

Use Breathing to Stay Present

Take a deep breath right now, making sure it goes deep into your belly. Shallow breathing that doesn't allow much oxygen to get into your body won't help. Shallow breathing deadens the senses, keeping you more in your head *thinking* rather than in your body *feeling*. When enough oxygen exists in your body, you can feel more sensations. Feeling enhances your ability to stay in the present moment.

Loosen your clothing, allowing yourself to breathe deeply into your belly. Keep this deep breathing going for as long as you want and feel yourself *in* the present moment.

Adding sound to your out breath allows any tension you're holding to release and dissipate. Let out a sound—a loud one—during your exhale. If your environment doesn't let you be loud, make a mental note to allow yourself that opportunity at a later time.

Expand your diaphragm as you breathe. Feel your breath opening your chest and your back. Breathe into all these spaces, allowing your body to completely relax. Hold your breath for a few seconds before letting it out.

Experiment with how you can use breathing to stay present and release tension at the same time.

I like to focus first on my exhale, pushing the last bit of air out of my body before beginning my inhale. Practicing yoga or using guided meditations, instructors ask participants to breathe *in* first. For a change, breathe *out* first.

When I focus on my exhale first, it allows me to better expel all the old breath from my body. I want to push the last bit of breath out to remove any impurities stored in my body. These pollutants stay in my body when I breathe in a shallow way or when I don't fully exhale, something that happens when I'm feeling scared and stressed.

I also find that pushing this breath out of my body during an exhale allows me to completely release any tension I feel. It also frees up space for my inhale to bring additional oxygen into my body. Alternating between expelling my breath evenly and slowly and expelling it quickly helps eliminate toxins in my body.

As I play with my breathing, I eventually want to make sure my exhale equals my inhale, which encourages balanced breathing. I check my breathing balance periodically by counting on my exhale and then making sure my inhale lasts for that same count. Equal breathing keeps me thriving, providing me with an invaluable technique to keep my body healthy and in equilibrium.

Try This Breathing Technique

Count this way on your exhale: 1,001, 1,002, 1,003, 1,004. Now on your inhale: 1,001, 1,002, 1,003, 1,004. Continue counting for several breaths until you can determine if that feels typical. Strive to feel a circular movement with your breath with no interruption between your exhale and your inhale. Envision one unbroken circle of air moving out of your lungs and nostrils and then back in again.

If breathing like this feels normal to you, chances are you already breathe in balance. If not, this could be a new technique to help bring your body back into balance.

When I first taught myself to breathe deeply on a regular basis, I wrote sticky note reminders and put them everywhere—on my computer screen, my car steering wheel, the bathroom mirror. I asked everyone I knew to remind me to breathe deeply, and I reminded others to breathe deeply, which helped me establish this new habit. For a while, I even featured the word BREATHE in big letters on my computer's screensaver. Deep breathing not only adds to one's health, it contributes to more enjoyment during sex because it increases the body's ability to feel.

Ask Your Man to Breathe With You

You may want to ask your man to help you remember to breathe deeply during your intimate time together, using the format I described when I asked Steve to ensure safety on our home. The conversation might go this way:

"Steve, I'd like to ask you a question. I want to talk with you about something important that will improve our sex life. It involves how I breathe during sex. When would be a good time to talk about this?"

"Let's talk about this right now." (Even though Steve wasn't initiating sex at this time, he still was interested in anything that might make our sex life better.)

"I'm reading this book, and it recommends that I breathe deeply during sex to increase the sensations in my body. I'd like you to remind me to breathe deeper when you notice that my breathing is short and quick. Would you be willing to do that?"

"Yes. Show me what short and quick looks like."

"It's almost like when I'm panting like a dog. (I hung my tongue out and panted, causing us both to laugh.) I know my breathing gets going faster when I'm sexually excited, so this can be kinda tricky. I want you to help me breathe deeply, even if I'm breathing faster. Does that make sense?"

"I think so."

"Would you be willing to share your understanding of what I'm asking?"

"You want me to make sure you breathe deeply during our intimate times together. This will help you feel more in your body. Is that right, and is there anything else?"

"That's correct, and there's nothing else. Are you willing to do that to help me?"

"Yes."

"How can I support you in doing this for me?"

"Remind me and give me feedback to help me learn more about how you breathe. Also, don't get mad at me if I don't do it right."

"I can do that. By doing this for me, Steve, you'll help me enjoy sex more and get more oxygen in my body. That means I'm happier and healthier. Thank you."

By reminding me to breathe deeply, it will also remind him to do the same. As Steve and I started breathing more consciously, we let each other know when one of us doesn't breathe deeply or evenly. We find our heart rate and blood pressure decreased, we feel more relaxed and connected to each other. Even if you're not in an intimate relationship with your man who has prostate cancer, discuss the importance of deep breathing with him.

One of the best ways to be intimate with your man involves breathing together, which may happen naturally anyway. I find it extra special when I'm aware of it. Consciously breathing with Steve keeps me in the present moment, preventing my mind from going places that could distract me from experiencing closeness. This type of breathing heightens my bond with Steve and helps me feel safe.

For different breathing exercises, I like the book *Conscious Breathing* by Gay Hendricks and video by Gay and Katie Hendricks called *Liberating Your Orgasm Reflex*. They explain and demonstrate how to breathe deeply and complement the breathing with pelvic exercises. The combination of these two methods opens up my body and relieves tension I feel in the moment.

Not only do these exercises provide long-lasting health benefits, I find them highly pleasurable. At times, doing them together provides comic relief for me and Steve. We enjoy laughing at our noises and movements. (If it doesn't work to do these exercises with your man, find a friend and ask her to practice them with you to add that fun dimension.)

Over time, I learned to move my breath throughout my entire body, which provided me with more freedom of movement, reduced my inhibitions, and helped me to stay focused on my body. Some women achieve orgasm through the simple act of breathing. What a beautiful example of self-care, no batteries required!

Learning how to breathe deeply opens the sexual satisfaction door wider so your man can satisfy you in different ways. This is important because much of the journey to physically thriving after prostate cancer involves looking at sex more creatively.

Satisfying you helps your man feel like he can "win" in the bedroom, which he may not feel often while being sexual after prostate cancer. Men pride themselves on satisfying their partners, so when you acquire new ways to experience more pleasure, it improves your man's self-confidence.

Add More Sounds

Consider incorporating more sound into your breathing during intimate times with your man. This may not feel comfortable to you, so I invite you to talk with him about it. Let him know you plan to experiment with ways you can feel more present in your body. Tell him you intend to make more sounds during sex, and that it may not come naturally to you. Let him know what he can do to support you and what it will provide for you. Play with your sounds, allowing your inhibitions to disappear as you create more safety in your relationship. Encouraging your man to make sounds too can make it easier for you to sound out your feelings.

Recently, Steve started making a snorting noise that brings a smile to my face. Picture a baby pig making a soft, contented sound as it drifts off to sleep after a big meal. I'm immediately attracted to him when he makes that sound.

Soon we found ourselves spontaneously kissing and making animal noises—the baaaaa sound like a sheep. I started making my award-winning duck noise that tickles my throat and makes Steve chuckle. (Yes, I once won a bottle of wine in an impromptu animal noise competition on the bus ride back after touring a Santa Barbara winery. Steve followed my quacking with his non-award winning gecko imitation—a sound I enjoy hearing.)

As our play continued and our passion increased, I was soon releasing the sound of "ham" (pronounced "haahhmmnng") that sometimes bursts out of my mouth during an orgasm. This sound relates to the Sanskrit word associated with the throat chakra. A chakra, often defined as an energy center, is founded in ancient Hindu texts. The sound "ham" resonated through my body, clearing my energy and causing me to feel completely present.

Our intimate time together continued as our breath slowed and we enjoyed lying next to each other. We practiced breathing alternately, so when Steve breathed in, I exhaled. After several minutes, our breathing merged together, we exhaled and inhaled together, completing our feeling of oneness.

Experiment with Your Breathing

Identify ways your breathing can help you stay present in each moment. Consider doing the following:

- Breathe deeply into your belly, expanding your diaphragm and loosening your clothing if needed.
- Focus on your exhale first, pushing all the air out of your lungs with a loud sound.
- Breathe in, holding your breath for a few seconds.
- Balance your breathing by making sure your inhale equals your exhale.
- Post notes all around, reminding you to breathe.
- Enjoy consciously breathing together with your man.
- Add fun sounds during intimate times.

Dancing

I love to dance around the house. Steve enjoys watching me and sometimes dances with me. Men appreciate it when women are happy, and most women "get happy" when they dance.

Dance provides me with increasing benefits the more I experiment with it. Like deep breathing, dancing moves energy throughout my entire body, allowing me to release tension and anxiety—both destroyers of great sex. The more I can eliminate them, the better I feel.

Despite taking dance classes over the years, I'm not a natural dancer and have trouble finding my rhythm. But that doesn't stop me from dancing! Because dancing helps me feel sexy and feminine, lightening my mood and giving my body a quick burst of energy, I consciously make it an essential part of my day.

What's more, dancing doesn't require much time and space. Even when I'm rushing through the day, I might dance a few steps in the restroom or move my body in the car in a dance-like way. I make it a priority to spread my energy throughout my body every day.

So I don't have to spend time searching for just the right music when I want to dance at home, I created a dance playlist on my computer using iTunes that includes my favorites. I also take note when a song plays in the background that arouses my body to move or causes my feet to tap. When possible, I add that song to my dance playlist.

Let your man know if you want to take dance classes. Because he might not understand what it brings to you, he could resent your time away from home. However, if he knows that dance helps you stay in your body and makes you a better partner for him, it's possible he'll *encourage* you to take classes.

> ## Vive la Dance!
>
> Want to make sure you take time to dance? Take dance classes!
>
> Belly dancing, for example, can be a fun and useful form of dance for women learning to thrive after prostate cancer. It moves the pelvic area, the part of the body where energy can get stuck if you don't enjoy sex regularly. In fact, many exercise classes provide a dance element that allows you to move your energy in healthy ways.
>
> Many women enjoy Zumba classes or classes that incorporate Latin, jazz, salsa, reggae, and swing dancing. (Search online to find a wide variety of options in your area.)

For Mother's Day last year, a friend received a series of dance classes from her husband and two sons. They knew that dancing made her happy, so they wanted to make sure she danced every week. If your man doesn't think of this, suggest it to him. You may have a friend who wants to thrive after prostate cancer or who just likes to dance. If so, take the classes together.

Often, couples find that taking dance classes together brings them closer to each other after prostate cancer. Although many men say they don't want to dance, claim they can't learn, and don't want to take the time (ever heard this?), mostly these comments come from a concern that they won't "win" in a dance class. Men want to win in all areas of life, so they won't set themselves up for failure. If they think they can't learn how to dance well or believe other men will be better dancers or doubt their woman will support them, they won't even try.

So You Want to Dance . . .

If you want to take dance classes with your man yet he resists, consider using the feedback method described earlier. Here's what the dialogue might be like:

"Excuse me, Steve. I'd like to share something that I'm excited about. When can we talk?"

"Can it wait until we have dinner in a few hours?"

"Sure, that will be fine."

"Remember that I wanted to share something with you that I'm excited about? Well, I was talking with a friend whose husband had his prostate removed a year ago. She said one of the best things they've done to improve their sex life is to take dancing lessons. She said she feels really happy when she's dancing, and they have great sex when they get home. Would you be willing to take dancing lessons with me?"

"How would that work?"

"I found a class for beginners that starts next Tuesday night. It lasts six weeks."

"I'd be willing to give it a try."

"Is there anything you need from me to attend these classes with me?"

"Just understand that I don't feel very comfortable dancing."

"Okay. Thank you for investing in our relationship. I feel really good about this."

Your objective is to help him understand what learning to dance will do for you (and thus him). Ask him if he can support you with this part of your healing process, and then look for ways to make sure he "wins."

Determine the type of dance your man might be able to learn more easily than others. Allow him to lead and gain confidence with this new skill. Compliment him often. Then compliment him some more, always with complete sincerity. A man has a fine-tuned BS meter and will know if you're not being truthful. Reinforcing your man's progress in learning a new skill will pave the way to getting your needs met. If he sees and believes that dancing brings you happiness, chances are he'll dedicate himself to learning this new skill.

On the other hand, if your man already loves dancing, determine what type of dance feels erotic to you, such as salsa or tango. Practice increasing the passion through dance, further spicing up your sex life. Make it the perfect start to a special evening. Dance together or separately. Touch each other or not. Experiment with which moves get you into your body. Stay present and connected with your man.

As a prostate cancer survivor who's supporting a brother, uncle, or friend rather than an intimate partner, still encourage him to dance the night away as a way to assist his healing process. He may take dance lessons with someone other than his intimate partner he feels safe with. Or you could suggest he take dance lessons on his own to surprise his wife or lover. Alternatively, he may want to take classes alone that add body movement like Tai chi, Qigong, Nia, or a martial art like Judo, Taekwondo, or Aikido.

If taking lessons doesn't appeal, he might experiment on his own to get his energy moving throughout his body, helping him feel more confident and alive. Remember the goal: to become more present in each moment. Dance, dance, dance!

Balancing Hormones

Because most men receive a prostate cancer diagnosis after age 50 and their significant others tend to be about that same age, women in intimate relationships with men being treated for prostate cancer can find their emotions affected by perimenopause, or early menopause. That's a full double whammy to deal with!

While I'm not a medical doctor, I know from experience (mine and my girlfriends') that female hormones can fluctuate a lot going through "the change." Add the stress of a prostate cancer diagnosis to the equation and what happens?

In my case, my hormonal changes caused night sweats and hot flashes. A small daily dose of bio-identical progesterone and estrogen quickly brought my hormones back into balance, helping me get a good night's sleep and no longer needing to wipe my sweaty upper lip while in meetings.

Stay Strong with Healthy Practices

Take advantage of the wealth of information available to guide you through this transitional time. Do all you can to stay strong with diet, exercise, and other healthy practices. Your man needs your strength to get him through his health crisis.

In addition, ask your man to get his hormones checked professionally to make sure his testosterone and other hormones are balanced and/or stabilized at a healthy level. Steve found his energy level increased after he started using a topical testosterone cream.

Sleeping Well

Why include sleep in this book about thriving after prostate cancer? Because sleep is an elixir essential to recovery and health, a fact proven by research posted at the website for the National Sleep Foundation (*www.NationalSleepFoundation.org*). I find my body requires more sleep than usual during stressful times. My body wants this extra sleep to process my emotions and because I may not sleep as well when I'm feeling worried and upset.

In November 2010, a global survey of more than 30,000 people in 23 countries commissioned by the Philips Center for Health and Well-Being showed that people in the U.S. have one of the highest rates of sleep deprivation. I'm definitely one of those people. I don't want sleep to interfere with the many things I love to do! That said, as increasingly more medical information indicates the health advantages of sleep, I intend to get the right amount and the right kind of sleep for my body. For me, that's about seven hours of uninterrupted sleep each night.

Getting enough sleep allows me to stay present and live life with less stress. When I'm tired, I'm often short-tempered (just ask Steve) and respond to difficult situations by snapping at Steve and getting angry at him over an incident that typically wouldn't bother me.

I can usually control how I express my anger with people I don't know well, but for those close to me—look out! What a terrible gift to give Steve!

Even more terrible is that I don't like myself when I lose my temper with people I love. I've observed that we relax more around those we know well, which typically enhances our relationships. Not so when we feel so comfortable that we react to situations in unhealthy ways with special people rather than taking a deep breath, counting to 10, or taking a self-imposed time-out.

I intend to treat those closest to me with my best behavior, giving them the gift of what they want to receive. When I don't, I'm given the opportunity to practice my apology skills and make the commitment to do better next time.

Getting enough rest lets me *respond* thoughtfully to situations instead of spontaneously *react* to them out of emotion. I'm able to understand others better and let compassion guide my actions. I'm kinder to myself and others. I'm sure you can add to this list of benefits when you feel well rested yourself.

Why Sleep? Let's Count the Benefits

Name all the benefits you receive from getting enough rest. As you realize the importance of sleep, you may be convinced to make sleep a higher priority than before. When you do that, you take control of your life rather than reacting to it.

Using a Neti Pot

As you work through your healing process, you may find your sinuses becoming stuffy or infected. Mine sure got that way. Years ago, when I felt terrible from a cold and sounded even worse, three friends in one week suggested I use something called a neti pot to clear my sinus cavities. A neti pot looks like a magical Aladdin's lamp or a small teapot.

Every day, I fill my neti pot with warm water and one-quarter teaspoon of salt. I turn my head to one side, insert the spout of the neti pot into one nostril, and allow the salt water to flow out my other nostril, clearing my sinuses in the process. I then tilt my head to the other side and pour water through my sinuses the other way. I often do two rounds of these clearings with one neti pot of water, allowing me to breathe easily all day.

Adding the use of a neti pot to my daily regime keeps me healthy. I recommend it to friends, and many of them find using it reduces sinus infections.

I went to the place where I purchase vitamins to buy a beautiful clay neti pot. Two days later, it broke when showering, raising a lot of concern about broken pottery on the shower floor. After that experience, I searched the Internet and discovered a plastic neti pot from SinuCleanse® I could buy at a drugstore. I actually use this neti pot every morning, and it accompanies me when I travel. I use it more often when I feel stuffiness in my nose or when I'm going through a difficult period.

When I tell people about it, some laugh and/or find the thought of putting water up their noses disgusting. I understand, although blowing my nose and sounding stuffed up can also be disgusting. I'd much rather do something that can help me feel healthy, even if it involves something gross.

Feeling Unattractive and Undesired

After Steve's diagnosis, he withdrew emotionally, and I couldn't find a way to reach him. We lived like roommates who didn't get upset (too often) when one of us ate the other one's food. We got along well with each other, we just didn't connect in ways other than household responsibilities and what each other did during the day.

Even after Steve's surgery, I couldn't reach him for three years. Periodically I'd erupt in anger over our lack of conversation about more meaningful topics and the disappearance of our sex life. This didn't help the situation; in fact, it harmed it, creating a larger chasm between us. The angrier I became, the more Steve withdrew. The more he withdrew, the angrier I became.

This change in our relationship wreaked havoc on my self-confidence. I fantasized about engaging in an affair or a one-night stand with some knight in shining armor. Before long, it became essential for me to find ways to feel attractive that wouldn't break up our relationship.

As noted earlier, Steve asked that I share his prostate cancer diagnosis and treatment with only a few individuals. I decided to share his lack of sexual interest in me with one person. That experience didn't provide any viable solutions, so I continued to hide my situation, suffering in silence. His withdrawal hurt so much that I struggled to figure out what to do.

Fortunately, the person I see for acupuncture treatments became a compassionate sounding board so I could express my thoughts and feelings when I really needed to. And fortunately, Steve felt okay with my talking about our relationship with her. She provided a comforting nonjudgmental acceptance, and her perspective offered me insights. Thank goodness for this welcome outlet.

Avoid Attacking Him

Take care to avoid attacking your man for his lack of sexual interest—a natural reaction of men in this situation. I suggest venting your feelings with medical providers, a counselor, or friends who can support you. When you get your frustrations out this way, you're in a more stable place to support your man's recovery, which will eventually support your own.

My New Best Friend

At various points during this period in my life, a vibrator became my best friend. I used it in private and didn't tell Steve about this activity. I'm not proud of that because I don't like hiding anything from him. But I didn't feel I could be open and straightforward during this time. I simply didn't know how to communicate my sexual needs and frustrations without attacking his masculinity and asking for a sex life that I didn't think he could provide. One that included intimacy and vulnerability that neither one of us was ready to offer.

In hindsight, I could have asked Steve for what I needed in a way he could understand and clearly stated the impact of his behavior on me. If I'd let him know how I felt, maybe we would have found ways for him to respond to help me feel better about myself and our relationship.

No question that Steve wanted me to be happy. Three long years after his surgery when we finally started to communicate our feelings to each other, I learned he was willing to help me in any way, including sexually.

Unfortunately, back then, I didn't know what to do and couldn't find any answers. I felt undesirable, unattractive and ignored as a woman. This rejection, whether real or perceived, hurt me deeply. It was a Catch-22: I wasn't sure he could regain interest in me sexually, and I didn't want him to feel like a failure if he couldn't.

How to Dialogue About Sex

If you find yourself not knowing what to say to get your needs met, consider using the request format modeled earlier to communicate

---

your desires to your man and find solutions. I wish I had initiated a dialogue that had sounded like this:

"Steve, I want to schedule some time to talk with you about something really important to me. Everything's okay, I just want to chat about how I'm feeling about sex."

"Could it wait until I get back from the gym?"

"Yes. When you get home, let's get something to drink, sit in our chairs and talk."

"It's been six months since my surgery. What about sex do you want to talk about?"

"I'm feeling unattractive and hurt because it feels like you don't want me sexually. I want you to know I'm not blaming you. I want you to initiate sex, helping me feel desired as a woman. Is that something you can do?"

"Probably not. I don't know what's going on, but I don't feel interested in sex, and I don't know what to do about it. Is there something else I can do?"

"I'm scared to initiate sex, as I don't know what it looks like any more. Are you okay if you don't have an orgasm?"

"I guess so. I'd like to please you and make sure you're happy. Would that help you?"

"We could try. If I initiate sex, will you be honest with me if it's not a good time for you? Also, will you think about how you can generate a sincere interest in sex?"

"Yes, I can do both. If you initiate sex, I'll either respond or let you know I'm not interested, in a nice way. I'll also give some thought to how I can become interested in sex again."

"Is there anything else I can do to support you with this?"

"Just give me some time."

"Okay. It's going to take me time to gather the courage to initiate sex. When we do, I know this will make me feel happier and more attractive as a woman. Thank you for being willing to support me with this."

Your goal in this dialogue? Let him know what you require as a woman and ask if he's willing and able to provide it for you. If he can't, try other avenues until you find something that helps. Your choices might include:

- Asking your girlfriends to compliment you on how you look.
- Use a vibrator, your hands, a Jacuzzi jet, or even a cucumber to enjoy an orgasm.
- Take a lap dance or pole dance class.
- Look inside for what you seek and then give it to yourself.
- Buy new lingerie.
- Take a bubble bath.

Don't give up too soon. Give both of you time to experiment with what will work for your relationship.

The Joy of Hearing Compliments

Hearing compliments from Steve would have made a difference to my self-confidence, although I didn't realize it at the time.

Ask For and Accept Compliments

If compliments will help you feel better as a woman and your man agrees to sincerely compliment you, accept it graciously. Soak in each full, juicy compliment even if it's subtle and a little awkward. Give him feedback about how good his compliment makes you feel and how much you appreciate his noticing. Avoid counter-productive responses such as, "You like this dress? I think I look fat in it," or "You didn't like this meal the last time I fixed it." Just say "Thank you." By reinforcing his positive behavior, you will keep the compliments coming—a bonus during this difficult time. Likewise, give *him* more compliments than you usually would. It's tough going for both of you.

Complimenting Steve in a sincere manner keeps me focused on what he does well, not the things that bother me about him. Now, I know that when I felt unattractive and undesired, such compliments would have shifted my attention from what *didn't* work in our relationship to what *did* work. I expect this shift in perspective would have lightened my load and perhaps changed the whole dynamic of our relationship at the time.

Based on my reading, I now understand that men often lose their desire for sex after treatment for prostate cancer. Not knowing that fact earlier caused me a lot of pain. Yet it makes sense. Because a man doesn't know how his sexual parts will work after treatment, he's likely afraid to find out.

Understanding your man's loss of desire and clearly communicating your needs can save you a lot of pain and frustration. Together, discover ways he can help you feel desired and attractive. Guide him along the way. Get his attention and make a statement before each idea you give him. That way, he knows how much it means to you. To avoid disappointment, be sure to obtain his agreement. Write your ideas for how you want to be treated on small pieces of paper and draw one out each day or week for him.

Here are a few suggestions:

- Notice how my earrings match my outfit.
- Comment on the color of my nail polish.
- Plant a lingering kiss on the back of my neck.
- How 'bout whistling at me when I walk in the room.

Add to this list in your journal or at the website Steve and I created: *www.SolutionsForIntimacy.com.*

If you find yourself supporting a woman in an intimate relationship with a man diagnosed with prostate cancer, use the information provided here as a guide to talk with her about her experience. Offer suggestions and help her find healthy ways to ensure she feels desirable and attractive.

If you support a man through recovery with whom you don't have an intimate relationship, help him become aware of what his partner may feel. Encourage him to talk about his feelings, letting him know that many men recovering from prostate cancer feel the same way. Delve into the next section for more ways to support him.

Balancing Female/Male Qualities

I felt quite confused about my role as a woman before, during, and after Steve's prostate cancer treatment. Unclear on how to best support him, I drifted toward a masculine role quite often. I took charge of situations, analyzed information, and went about life in a logical manner. I became harder, seemingly losing many of my feminine qualities like creativity, softness, and compassion that had enhanced our relationship in the past. Head down, I lived in survival mode yet extremely out of balance. In hindsight, that didn't serve me or our relationship well at all. Learning to become more feminine and reducing my masculine behaviors allowed me to fulfill an important part of my own recovery process.

During this time, Steve lost his zest for life. He worked more and traveled away from home almost every week. Home alone, I became the one to take care of all household matters, even those he typically handled like the yard service. Meanwhile, he seemed to withdraw even more into himself. Now I understand that he didn't know what else to do, and this was a safety mechanism for him. If my feminine qualities of compassion and nurturing prevailed at this time, I believe our recovery would have occurred sooner.

For years, I didn't know much about how feminine and masculine qualities worked within me and within a relationship. I didn't realize that every human contains aspects of both. Since then, I've learned that feminine qualities are often associated with the right side of the brain and with feelings and intuition. Conversely, masculine qualities are associated primarily with the left side of the brain and with thinking and logic. Over time, I discovered that, for my life and my relationships to thrive, I had to put the feminine and masculine qualities within me into balance.

I also needed to discern when to use feminine behaviors and when more masculine traits were appropriate. Neither is better or worse than the other; both qualities provide value for either men or women at certain times. For example, in emotional situations like prostate cancer, my masculine quality of analysis allows me to focus on continued treatment options. Similarly, my masculine ability to take charge and lead causes me to initiate sex when Steve doesn't rise to the occasion.

For years, I lived under the misconception that "real" men don't exhibit feminine qualities. Ironically, I also believed that using masculine qualities would ensure success for me, even though I'm a woman. This belief was essentially a result of our culture, which in most cases, rewards masculine aspects more than feminine ones, regardless of the gender of the individual.

Case in point: I struggled as a woman working in business because the world of work valued masculine qualities like stability, competition, and ambition over feminine qualities such as beauty, sensitivity, and compassion. How could I succeed in business without becoming more like a man? I couldn't see how, yet I wanted to succeed in that world. So I adopted analytical, assertive, so-called masculine qualities and, in retrospect, realized I devalued my feminine side—my creativity, intuition, and nurturing.

> If your life path and natural tendencies have developed your feminine qualities more than your masculine ones, you may not relate to my experience of living in a traditionally masculine role. If your nurturing, creative skills dominate, you might be out of balance if you haven't developed the so-called masculine qualities of planning and implementing. The mix of these qualities differs for each individual, so honor your process of what works to achieve balance for you.

For example, as a CPA, I used my left-brain talents with efficiency. I succeeded when my logical mind analyzed a problem and then figured out and implemented a solution. I received pay raises for this behavior, rewarding me for my assertive decision-making. No one encouraged me to use compassion and intuition at work.

Yet all this time, I felt out of balance, ignoring a host of my abilities. My masculine qualities had overtaken me. As I studied ways to thrive after prostate cancer, I became aware that cultivating my femininity would elevate my healing to a new level. As a side benefit, it also assisted Steve's healing process.

My work life benefited also through increased productivity and profits. Working with other team members, we created a vision board to depict our desired office space. It provided hidden gems to guide us to make sure we offered a fun, welcoming environment with color. The team at work developed trust and sincerity skills through training in authenticity and effective feedback techniques.

Feminine and Masculine Qualities

What are feminine and masculine qualities, or female and male energies? Read through this partial list and determine which ones you relate to well. Are you balanced with both of these energies or, like me, do you gravitate to one side of the chart more than the other?

Feminine Qualities	Masculine Qualities
Animated	Analytical
Colorful	Cool
Delicate	Logical
Gentle	Objective
Intuitive	Orderly
Joyful	Protective
Nurturing	Stable
Still	Strong

At a conference I attended a few months before this book's publication, author and thought-leader Richard Florida noted that feminine qualities such as creativity and social skills are keys for the future. A Catalyst Inc. study published in 2007 suggests that corporations with female representation on its board of directors out perform corporations without female representation.

As I studied and developed more feminine qualities within myself, I tuned into knowing when to use each one. My moment of discovery occurred when I reviewed feedback from participants in a corporate leadership class Steve and I taught together. The attendees enjoyed how well we worked together. As I contemplated this information, I discovered that Steve uses mostly masculine qualities when he teaches. I had brought more feminine qualities to the classroom without realizing it. Because of this dynamic, we established a balance that was noticed and appreciated by the participants.

After this discovery, I consciously started focusing on ways to balance Steve's masculine qualities. I offset his stability with more animation and counterbalanced his coolness by meeting the participants. After class, though, I found it helpful to make sure I used some of my masculine qualities. I took the lead with dinner reservations and packed away the classroom materials.

When I feel off-kilter, I go to my list of qualities to determine which ones will help me feel more balanced. Then I decide what I require to move myself back into balance and make adjustments.

If you have a sense that you might be out of balance, pick one or two qualities to develop. Ask someone who embodies the desired quality well to give suggestions. Read up on ways to acquire that quality. You may also discover, like I did, that reducing qualities that might dominate in your life can also bring you back into balance.

For example, if you find yourself living an orderly routine, drive to work a different way, pay bills at night instead of in the morning, and go to the left side of the grocery store for a change instead of going right to the produce section first.

As you understand the differences between feminine and masculine qualities and learn how to navigate between them within a relationship, watch your life move from just surviving to thriving.

✳ ✳ ✳

At this point, decide which qualities your man can help you with to bring more balance into your relationship, then ask for his assistance. Using the request format, your conversation might look like this:

"Steve, may I interrupt you for just a minute? I want to arrange a time to share something important that I've not mentioned before. I want you to help me use my feminine qualities more. When would be a good time to talk about this?"

"In about thirty minutes after I finish updating this computer software."

"I had a big aha moment today, Steve, about something that will create more balance in our relationship. If I bring more feminine qualities into our life, we can build on your skills of analyzing and bringing objectivity to situations. Would you be willing to do that?"

"I think so. What do you mean?"

"When we meet with our financial planner next week, I'd like you to take the lead and ask the tough questions. You're very good at that. I want to be less active, checking inside with my intuition by tuning into my feelings about our investment decisions. I also want to bring my feminine quality of sharing to the meeting, so I'll ask about his family and vacation plans. What do you think about that plan?"

"That will work. I'm not happy with some of the investment returns and don't understand one of his recommendations. How do I know when you want to talk about your feelings?"

"You can allow me to talk when I'm ready. Sometimes I don't feel heard because my voice is soft."

"Cindie, can you put your hand on my arm or something like that when you're ready to talk?"

"Yes, I'll do that. Can you please summarize your understanding of how you can help me use more of my feminine qualities during our meeting this week?"

"You want me to take the lead and ask the hard questions. You'll handle the soft stuff that I'm not really good at, like small talk. If I don't allow you to talk, you'll touch me to get my attention when you have something to say. Is that right, Cindie?"

"Yes. Are you willing to do that to help me?"

"Yes."

"Steve, is there anything else I can do to support you in doing this for me?"

"No. I can do this at other times, also, if you help me understand how and don't get mad at me if I don't do it right."

"Thank you, Steve. As we get better at this, I will feel happier and closer to you. Thank you for giving me this gift."

Becoming More Feminine

Not surprisingly, men question their masculinity during their recovery from prostate cancer. Women who are aware of this possibility can provide opportunities to help their men boost their masculine qualities. How? By enhancing their feminine qualities as listed.

Because I related more strongly to masculine qualities throughout my adult life, this activity challenged me. Finally, I enlisted the qualities of focus and planning to gain more feminine qualities. Isn't that ironic? I set goals to become more feminine and used my masculine qualities to achieve them. By the way, this also helped my inner male feel safe by honoring his gifts in this way.

How I became more feminine might sound funny to you. In fact, I'm smiling as I write about them because they sound funny to *me* now. But here's what I did.

First off, I started wearing skirts. This allowed me to become more aware of my body and how it felt. Some women switch from taking showers to taking more baths as a ritual to feel good. I started allowing men to open doors for me, and I began asking others to assist me with projects that I didn't find easy to do. Over time, applying awareness and effort, I could feel myself becoming a softer, warmer, and more nurturing human being.

Because feminine qualities include compassion and receptivity, I studied ways to bring these aspects into my daily life. I allowed myself to develop my intuition, although I still called it my "gut instinct" in most business situations. In the process of changing, I let my happiness out and allowed my tears of sadness to show—something new for me.

By learning to become more feminine, guess what? I experienced more of my human potential. Over time, I was able to balance the masculine and feminine energies in my body, allowing more aspects of myself to emerge in diverse ways. The more I got to know myself, the more I could bring this expanded self to my relationship with Steve and others.

In my situation, I could see how the masculine roles suit Steve well, but unfortunately, as I reflect on our prostate cancer journey, I didn't allow him to take these roles as much as I might have. By taking over so much, I denied him the opportunity to feel successful, in charge of situations, and contributing to our life together.

Indeed, I found it easier to use a vibrator by myself than to initiate sex. If he didn't have a preference for when we ate dinner, I just planned a time by myself. We went our separate ways with our investments, as I wasn't ready to listen to his ideas. In hindsight, I see I could have brought my feminine quality of compassion to the relationship, recognizing his hesitancy about sex. By waiting for him to make a decision about dinner, he could have been encouraged to participate in our lives more often. If I had been more cooperative and valued the feminine characteristic of sharing, we could have collaborated on our investments sooner. I believe he wanted to participate in all these ways. Like me, he didn't have the skills at the time.

Little did I know that by helping *so much*, I was doing harm! When Steve didn't feel confident about himself, he couldn't feel attracted to me, causing me not to feel confident about myself. It created a downward spiral that didn't resolve itself until I brought a balance of the male and female qualities into our relationship.

Today, I continue to focus on developing my softer feminine side and using my creativity more fully. This gives Steve more room to use his masculine strengths, a true win-win for both of us. His strong male side can get things done; my role is to make suggestions and get out of the way, allowing him to go into action. For example, while writing this book, I asked him to help by creating a website and getting ready to sell it online.

Previously, I probably would have attempted to do all of these things by myself.

Regain Sense of Masculinity

Review the list of feminine/masculine qualities noted earlier, then apply the intention of supporting your man to develop the qualities that can assist him to regain his sense of masculinity after prostate cancer. Determine what he does well and encourage him to thrive in those areas.

Did prostate cancer cause your man to move *more* into his masculine side? If so, he may require your support to use more of his feminine qualities. Refer to the list of masculine and feminine qualities and determine how to assist him in bringing his qualities into balance. Bonus: Doing so will also add balance to your relationship.

You can train yourself, as I did, to move in and out of whatever quality best serves a situation and other people. Perhaps you experience what's called unconscious competence, which means you can already do something (e.g., drive a car) but aren't aware of it. By understanding the concept more thoroughly and realizing you already have this ability to be flexible, you move into conscious competence (e.g., take driving lessons to improve your skill). From there, your heightened awareness of the skill allows you to further develop it.

Our goal? To live a life that thrives—both of us. When we travel together, I'm much better now at allowing him to take the lead. He confidently makes adjustments when our flight times change, his alertness allow us to know when a gate changes and his planning ahead allows us to know how to best connect to our next flight with ease.

I'm also giving up control over the planning of a major trip, something I haven't done before. Instead, I'm allowing my creative feminine side to make suggestions to Steve as to locations and desired hotel qualities. He has found some delightful properties for us to experience in the South Pacific. He's using his masculine analytical skills to find unique flight plans to conserve our money and time. Another bonus in this cooperative approach is the excitement and ownership I sense he finds from his involvement.

Understanding Our Masculine Side

Numerous books describe the complicated relationship between the feminine and masculine qualities within us. The "other side" of us (male if we are female, female if we are male) has been called our shadow side, our divided self, or our invisible partner. The more we can bring light to our dark side, acknowledge our shadow, and integrate it into our lives, the more balanced and whole our life becomes. When we learn how to reveal all parts of ourselves, we become more self-aware and conscious of our actions.

Carl Jung, renowned Swiss psychiatrist, proposed that a woman contains a man within her, and she must create a positive relationship with this man to establish beneficial relationships with other men. The opposite holds true for men whom Jung believed to have an inner female.

Bringing all aspects of our being to the light—balancing our masculine and feminine qualities—leads to healthier relationships. When we balance ourselves in this way, we eliminate projecting hidden aspects of ourselves onto others. We no longer search to fill what we mistakenly believe are holes in ourselves. Instead, we bring all of our being to each relationship, further enhancing our lives.

I learned about the dark side of my male through The Sedona Intensive, a personal transformation program for releasing chronic and unwanted patterns. Albert Gaulden, the program's founder, adapted Jung's concept of the shadow to produce a meditation for becoming acquainted with an individual's "shadow" and eventually integrate it.

When I first started using this meditation, I couldn't even look at my shadow. Unbelievable as it may seem, I would shake in fear of this masculine part of me.

With Albert's assistance, I named my male shadow Charlie. Personifying this part of me allowed me to begin a healthy relationship with him. Even though I don't fully understand all the theory and psychology behind this approach, all I needed for my healing was to get to know Charlie, to understand him.

I discovered that Charlie, in a sense, took over my life when I was a child. Like many of you, events in my early life caused me to feel unsafe. Charlie, my masculine side, took charge to protect me.

I hid my hurt feelings, toughening my soft feminine side. I didn't express myself, afraid that what I said would cause an angry response. I avoided showing any weakness, as strength was rewarded in my childhood.

Through several sessions with Albert and a psychologist, I confirmed that Charlie started running my life when I was a little girl. This masculine side of me took over when he felt I needed protection during certain situations that occurred during my childhood. It continued to protect me as I moved into adulthood.

As I worked through this realization, I began to understand why Charlie ran my life for so long—that is, he had become activated to keep me safe. The solution? To establish a relationship with him so I could have a balanced relationship with myself and a solid relationship with Steve.

After about three weeks, I overcame my fear of Charlie and started talking with him during the meditation. With Albert's voice instructing me during the meditation, I created a room with a glass coffee table in between two contemporary chairs. On the table, I imagined a vanilla candle calming the atmosphere and a vase of colorful flowers lightening the mood.

Eventually, when I greeted Charlie in this room, I gave him a big hug. I guided him to a chair and sat across from him. Our conversations went something like this:

"Charlie, I'm a big girl now and live in a safe environment. I really value all you did to protect me as a little girl. I also appreciate the masculine qualities you enabled me to hone like courage, independence and stability. Those qualities served me very well in business and in other parts of my life. I know you did what you thought was best for me.

"I no longer need your protection, although I will ask for it if I do. Now it's time for me to develop other skills that are important to me as a woman. These are more feminine skills like compassion, creativity and intuition. I've kept these qualities hidden for many years. Can you support me in this way?"

In my meditative state, I heard Charlie say, "Yes, I understand. I will always be here for you, and it's important that you keep reassuring me that you are safe. I may find it difficult to step aside, especially if I believe you are in danger." I thanked Charlie and completed the remainder of the meditation.

In one month, my connection with Charlie let me establish a more well-rounded and aware relationship with myself. I knew I had made progress during a conversation Steve and I had about a home he wanted to purchase in Sedona, Arizona. Early in the conversation, he mentioned his desire for granite counter tops, taking out a wall, and replacing the flooring.

Immediately, Charlie stepped into the conversation for me. Before I knew it, I was saying, through Charlie's voice, that I didn't want a major financial expense right now. I accused Steve of being insensitive to our savings goals. The anger in my voice and my inability to listen to Steve caused me to realize what was happening. I asked for a time-out.

I took a deep breath. This wasn't Cindie talking. It was Charlie. So I started having a chat with Charlie, letting him know that Steve and I were only brainstorming about the home purchase. I told him that I wanted to find out more from Steve in a reasonable manner and promised not to make any decisions that would harm me. I thanked Charlie for wanting to keep me from making a financial mistake and asked him to support me while I talked with Steve about his desires.

I apologized to Steve, sharing with him my discovery that Charlie had taken over, wanting to keep me safe. Steve and I continued the conversation, with me asking questions and listening to him dream about remodeling the house. After a while, Steve commented that he didn't think it was a good idea to purchase the property.

Because I recognized Charlie's voice quickly in this conversation, I was able to calm his fears and continue a productive conversation with Steve. This situation allowed me to feel more confident in my ability to recognize when my masculine side wants to take over, allowing me the opportunity to break a pattern and have a healthy exchange with Steve.

Explore Your Own Shadow Side

Explore ways you can integrate your shadow, your divided self—an unrecognized part of you that has more power than you want to give it. Therapists can assist you with this process. So can books and other written resources. For a start, see the Resources section at the end of this book.

Most important of all, keep your focus on becoming a balanced, feminine, authentic woman who is destined to thrive after prostate cancer.

Balancing Feminine and Masculine Qualities in the Bedroom

With my new focus, it didn't take much to realize that understanding female and male qualities could improve my sex life—something that applies to anyone, not only survivors of prostate cancer.

Steve and I began exploring our roles in the bedroom about two years after his diagnosis. We learned that allowing each of us to play different parts added a new dimension. I don't mean performing roles of different characters, although some couples find that enjoyable. I'm referring to our female and male roles.

For example, in our play, Steve and I mixed up who brings feminine qualities to the bedroom and who brings masculine qualities for variety and creativity. As we got better at "pretending" to play a certain role, it occurred naturally. In the beginning, though, we spent time talking and making sure we agreed on what role each of us would play.

Time to Take the Lead in the Bedroom

In many relationships, the man often plays more of the masculine role and initiates sex more frequently than the woman. After prostate cancer, this may not happen. Your man's confidence may be shaken, and he may not believe he can "win" in the bedroom. It could be time for you to take the lead and play the masculine role, initiating sex more often than you usually would.

This can be daunting if you don't have the skill set or the desire to "play" an assertive role. However, as you view sex in a whole new way, learning additional skills can assist with your own healing process and move you from surviving to thriving.

This happened to me, although I admit neither one of us initiated sex very often even before prostate cancer. When I discovered my desire for a healthy sex life and a thriving marriage, I accepted the fact that I would take the role of initiating sex more frequently than Steve did—and certainly more frequently than I had done before. At first, I didn't want to take on that role, but my desire for a better sex life overcame my fears. Bonus: My decision brought up the self-doubt I'd frequently felt during my younger years—also feeling insecure, uncertain, even embarrassed, too.

As I initiated sex more often, I wondered how I looked and realized how terrible I would feel if I couldn't reach an orgasm. In fact, I contemplated faking an orgasm to save Steve from feeling as if he'd failed to satisfy me in the traditional sense.

And I worried. What might happen if Steve rejected me and didn't want sex? Looking back, I remembered experiencing rejection in my younger years. I recalled my wounded feelings when a man I wanted didn't want me.

I didn't sense Steve desired me after his surgery. The typical hardness I sometimes felt next to me before surgery didn't appear. I didn't know how to approach him when we didn't know what sex looked like post-surgery. Clearly my skills weren't developed enough yet.

List Your Fears

Do you resist initiating sex? I invite you to add to the list of fears noted here. Alternatively, you can change them to what causes you to not want to take this more masculine role in the bedroom. Pay attention. Do you deal with fears like these?

- Rejection because your man is not showing an interest in you sexually.
- Showing your naked body because your thighs are too big, your breasts sag, you don't like your stretch marks, etc. The concerns about your body can go on and on.
- Not knowing how to make love when an erection doesn't occur or if your man has difficulty getting it up.
- Hurting your man physically after his recent surgery.
- Your vagina being too dry due to menopause or another cause.

On the flip side, here's what felt wonderful. Once I became aware of my fears, I could address them and share them with a handful of people to help me move past them. I could talk with Steve more openly. Thankfully, I could ask him to assist me in changing my behaviors of the past.

As I learned to live more in the present, these fears dissipated naturally. When I didn't project what might happen, it became easier for me to do new things because I didn't worry about failure or rejection. Here's the biggie: *I decided it didn't matter if I achieved an orgasm.*

In addition, when I didn't allow myself to think about uncomfortable experiences from my past, I summoned up more courage than ever before. That helped me move beyond my fears as I experienced the present moment and left the baggage of my past by the wayside.

From the Man's Point of View

Many men don't know what to do when they can't obtain an erection easily, so it often falls to the woman to figure out what sex looks like in this new world. Plus many men can't imagine sex without ejaculation, so they avoid sex altogether. There's more to sex than a hard penis; it's called foreplay. He may not know how satisfying touch and kissing can be, so taking the lead would help.

For a man to take a pill, use a pump, or inject a drug into his penis to obtain an erection requires planning, extra work, and new skills. It also raises the risk of failure. Your man may be thinking, "What if the pill doesn't work? . . . What if the shot hurts? . . . I want spontaneity . . . . This is too much trouble."

Generally speaking, if men don't know the rules of the new game, they simply decide not to play. Thus, women must learn the rules if we want to play the game. We must create an environment in which both of us can win.

Sex is personal and important to human beings. If we've had negative experiences with sex, it may not seem that important, and in fact, prostate cancer may bring relief from any feeling of obligation to have intercourse. However, let's consider the benefits sex offers to a couple and to us as women.

For all of us, sex can enhance feelings of love and joy. It connects us to our most authentic self, to our man and to something sacred, even divine. It causes us to transcend our physical body, satisfying our soul's desire for wholeness. Sexual intimacy allows us to escape our ego, surrender our expectations, and experience true freedom. It brings extra meaning to our relationship because, through sex, we share a part of ourselves that we don't share with anyone else. Remember, too, that sex brings about more vibrant health, so let's allow that fact to motivate us.

Take Charge of Your Sex Life

As a woman in the aftermath of your man's prostate cancer, you have the opportunity to take charge and create the sex life of your dreams. Offered a blank canvas, you can paint whatever picture you desire using your creative feminine gentleness and your masculine focus.

Apply the communication technique used throughout this book to engage your man. A conversation might sound like this:

"Steve, I want to talk about ways to jump-start our sex life. I know I haven't been a very good partner in this area, and I have some ideas of how I can do things differently. When would you be free to talk?"

"Let's talk now. I'm very interested in this topic!"

"Well, this is a bit difficult, so please put your arm around me so I feel safer. For some reason, I'm embarrassed to tell you what I really want from our sex life. (Take a deep breath here.) I really enjoy it when you rub lotion all over my body, kissing me along the way, especially kissing between my toes. I get really excited with this slow, soft way of making love. If it feels right, I love reaching an orgasm from oral sex, although I don't want to feel pressured to have to come. Does that make sense?"

"Yes, you want me to spend time focusing on your body by being gentle and attentive. You love oral sex, although you don't want to feel forced to have an orgasm. Am I right?"

"Yes. Also, Steve, I read about men who can experience an orgasm without an erection. It's done through the movement of energy, or something like that, and I'd like us to spend more time touching you to see if we can figure out how it works. I don't want either one of us to feel pressured in the process, though. It would help if we just experiment and play with new techniques to see what we like."

"I can do that. It sounds pretty weird, but I miss our sex life, and I miss having orgasms. If you will take the initiative, I'll follow along."

"Okay. And Steve, you can help me by being open to my taking the lead. This is new to me. Also, please talk with me during sex. That will help me know if what I'm doing feels good to you."

"Sure. I want you to talk with me, too. I'm feeling new at this also, so I need your feedback."

"Please share your understanding of this part of our conversation, letting me know if there's anything else I can do to support you."

"You want me to see if I can have an orgasm in a new way and try different things to see what works. I will be open to your initiating sex and tell you how I'm feeling, Cindie. You're going to do the same."

"Thank you, Steve. I know we can learn together what sex looks like after prostate cancer. I will enjoy improving our connection and having fun with our sex life."

After a conversation like this, invite him to participate in a way that will help him feel good about himself and learn how to win at this new game of sex after prostate cancer.

Achieving Intimacy with Yourself

Some teachers say, "To become intimate with another, you must become intimate with yourself." Others elaborate with, "Intimacy means Into Me See," noting the importance of looking inside to get to know ourselves at a deeper level. Often people view intimacy from a spiritual or emotional perspective. To thrive after prostate cancer, I found it important to also know myself better physically.

Searching for books, classes, Internet sites, and videos can teach us how to explore our bodies and discover what gives us pleasure in the privacy of our homes. Coaches and therapists can also guide us on this path to discovering what works to become physically intimate. Let me share what worked for me and what didn't.

Intimacy Parties

Soon after Steve had his prostate removed, a friend invited me to a gathering called an intimacy party. Curious, I discovered that only female guests would attend, and we could learn about and purchase items to enhance our sex lives. I hadn't been to this type of party before and walked in with an open mind. Or so I thought.

In truth, I felt uncomfortable because I hadn't shared Steve's recent prostate-free situation with anyone. With more than 20 women there, we enjoyed an abundance of alcoholic drinks, delicious food, and conversation about sex. Much of that conversation centered on erections and ejaculation. We shared techniques to help men last longer and made jokes about premature ejaculation. A few times, I caught myself close to tears because I knew ejaculation wouldn't be a part of my future. At that point, I didn't know if an erection would be either.

Yet despite my fears of the unknown and keeping my secret to myself, I enjoyed the party. I learned a lot about myself from talking with the others and the person selling the products. I left inspired by the other women who took ownership of their sexual fulfillment by taking the lead in their relationships. Plus I learned that I already had many of the tools I needed to enjoy a hot sex life; I just hadn't made using them a priority.

I knew how my body worked, I was familiar with vibrators, and I had a great imagination—something I discovered when I set out to write my erotic novel. I also had a man in my life. Many of the women at the party didn't and were searching for the right partner. I left with a new vibrator, a rabbit hair mitt, and some lotions with pheromones and flavors. (A pheromone is a chemical compound that some believe attracts the opposite sex.)

When the box of the products I ordered arrived, Steve and I unpacked it with excitement. We laughed at the descriptions and in talking about our new toys, we enjoyed a new type of intimacy together. This actually helped Steve see sex in a new light. I was happy I had taken the more masculine role and initiated the opportunity for us to learn together. Sure, it felt risky to me, yet afterward, I realized I'd gained a new sense of self-confidence.

Intimacy parties encourage women to take charge of their sexual fulfillment, although they're only a beginning. I, for one, required more training to fully accept that I'm responsible for my sexual fulfillment. I still wanted to lay this responsibility on Steve.

Over time, though, I experimented, learned about my body, and acquired new skills. I knew this process would keep me healthy—and keep my relationship with Steve fun and vibrant.

Pole Dancing

I had heard talk about pole dancing but didn't think a woman in her 50s would be a candidate to learn it. However—surprise! I ended up pole dancing on two occasions and will probably take classes in the future. Pre-prostate cancer, learning about pole dancing never entered my mind! Post-prostate cancer, I became more accepting of new experiences—an open-mindedness essential to learning how to thrive in my new life.

My first experience with pole dancing was instigated by a friend who was celebrating her 40th birthday. Believing in the importance of women getting to know their sexuality and increasing their self-confidence, she invited a former stripper to teach her female guests some new skills. What a great idea and gift from this friend—although I didn't think so at first! I felt scared. At age 50, not only was I one of the oldest women at the party, I didn't have any stripper heels like the others, and I didn't own anything sexy to wear.

Regardless of these disadvantages, though, I thoroughly enjoyed it. Before class, "Gloria," who taught the pole dancing, looked like all the other women. When she switched to her stripper persona, though, I saw an amazing transformation as she expertly engaged her feminine power. I immediately knew I could learn a lot from her.

Gloria taught us to love our bodies no matter what they looked like. As we learned moves on the pole, a new sense of confidence emerged. I enjoyed watching the others become more powerful. Before long, I began moving more comfortably in my body. During this time together, I laughed and was finally able to get over myself. After all, the other women felt just as self-conscious as I did. We agreed to support each other no matter who fell off their high heels or moved clumsily on the pole. I knew only one person at the beginning of the class, but by the end, we hugged and celebrated our newfound friendships—*and* our new sexual confidence.

Later that year, I took a half-day class to learn a pole dance routine. Once again, I was one of the oldest women in the class. It didn't matter, though, as the instructor typically provides support to women of all ages, sizes, and abilities. She taught us to feel our power and own our life force. I bought knee pads in preparation for the class, took along my highest heels (which weren't very high), and showed up with the intention to learn more about my sexuality.

During both of these pole dancing experiences, I discovered the value of staying present. By staying focused on my body and not living in my head, I could discover more about myself. My real power resides in the moment—and in my body. As I listen to what my body says, I allow its inklings to guide me. My head supports the process by allowing my body to share its desires, then figuring out ways to implement those desires. My biggest discovery? I had eliminated my tendency to overanalyze situations and worry. Becoming present in my body was the key.

Lap Dancing

As I explored new activities, my body suggested it might enjoy seeing how it feels to perform a lap dance. My head enrolled me in two different classes six months apart. As in my pole dancing classes, the instructor shared her patience and encouragement with us all and supported me, this woman of 50 plus who isn't a naturally gifted dancer. This time, though, I wasn't the oldest person in the class. Apparently, women of all ages have an appetite for learning how to lap dance.

Once again I felt challenged. To learn the dance moves and later perform them, I completely needed to stay in my body and out of my head—striving to feel sexy regardless of what my thighs look like or how I look compared to other women. Breathing helped; so did laughing a lot.

In addition, I enjoyed watching women who might not be considered sexy get into their bodies and discover their inner sex goddess. One of the women who practiced with me weighed 50 pounds more than her ideal weight. I watched with awe as she carried herself with pride and learned the dance moves a lot faster than I did. After class, we clearly walked taller, eyes sparkling with a fresh feeling of self-confidence.

I never did perform the first lap dance I learned for Steve, although I practiced it a number of times by myself. Back then, he didn't seem interested in this new part of my life. But since that time, I've understood that many men lack interest in sex after prostate cancer treatment. Indeed, even my *own* courage and desire for an improved sex life took time to evolve. Yet, as I enhanced my own sexuality, I gradually built up my desire for a sexual relationship with Steve, and eventually he reciprocated.

Yes, I did perform the second lap dance I learned for Steve—twice! One afternoon, I slipped into my Santa Baby costume, cranked up the volume of this Christmas tune, and felt sexy and in-charge of my life as I followed all the steps of the three-minute dance. While Steve enjoyed this performance, I got the most satisfaction out of how I took charge of my sexuality. With pride, I learned more about myself, owned my feminine power, and mustered the courage to do something difficult.

Find Your Power through Movement

Consider taking pole dancing or lap dancing lessons, either alone or with a friend. Find an instructor who uses this type of teaching to help women find their own power. Make sure the instructor focuses on you, as a woman keen to express her sexuality, not on how to find a man or keep one happy.

If you can't find an instructor, obtain a DVD to teach you. Watch it alone or make your learning session a party with several friends. Laugh and enjoy becoming intimate with yourself. This type of training can provide you much joy and courage to live your life as a thriving woman. A whole new world can open up to you.

Sex Shops

What about visiting sex shops? Before you say "no way," allow me to share my perspective about this activity. For many women, shopping offers the opportunity to be feminine, spend time with friends, and get lost in the moment. Most women, though, don't go shopping in a sex shop. I grew up believing that only perverts frequented these places, and that nice girls would never consider entering such a store. If I did go inside, I certainly didn't want anyone to see me. Over the years, I have run into a shop, bought a vibrator, and rushed out. A few of the places I went were dark and a bit scary—not anywhere I wanted to hang out.

While vacationing in Maine a year before Steve's diagnosis, he and I wandered down a street full of shops. One shop looked fun, so we went in to explore and discovered adult merchandise—right in this well-lit place located in the middle of a typical shopping area.

Surprised and a bit shocked, we did browse and ask questions. The staff person answered my questions patiently, and we kept asking about different items. I felt safe, had fun, and didn't feel uncomfortable. This opened my mind to the possibilities this type of merchandise could provide to help improve my sex life.

Unfortunately, the novelty of the dolphin-shaped vibrator we bought wore off, and we didn't yet have the skills to move past our fears of intimacy. I kept using the Smartballs I bought, though. (This product from Fun Factory can increase vaginal muscle tone and pleasure. YouTube has some educational videos that describe the benefits of Smartballs and how to use them.)

It took a while for me to get over my fear and the perceived stigma of going into an adult merchandise store on a regular basis. In fact, I feel sad that it took an experience with prostate cancer for me to get over my "issues" about this and give myself permission to explore the options these types of products provide.

These days, I sometimes go into these romantic accessory shops alone, spending all the time I want exploring the various sections of the store. Other times, Steve joins me and we check out the merchandise together. We occasionally browse for these types of products online, although I think it's more fun to see the variety first hand.

I also enjoy looking at sexy clothing, although I don't buy much of it. Perusing the titillating movie titles and pictures brings me ideas that I add to my ever-expanding knowledge base. And I love smelling the many fragrances that light up my senses in the lotions and oils section.

When I go to one of these shops with Steve or with friends, we giggle at something that seems ludicrous and ask each other, "Who would use this?" Stretching our imaginations, we like to guess how certain products could be used. We laugh a lot, appreciate the staff members who patiently answer questions, and then decide what to buy.

Books and Films about Sex

Books about sex provide a wealth of knowledge for women. In offering ideas and permission, they can also inspire creativity and exploration. Romance novels, for example, can boost feelings of sexiness.

I actually *wrote* an erotic novel soon after Steve's diagnosis. It just started coming out, which surprised me. Writing it gave me a great deal of pleasure and occupied my mind during that depressing time. Escaping into an exciting fantasy world actually helped me release a lot of stress. Looking back, I see I used writing as another way to avoid my fear of intimacy with myself and with Steve. It distracted me from looking at my life and our relationship.

My erotic novel hasn't been completed, and Steve is the only one who's read it. My close friends say they'd much rather read *that* book than the two personal growth books I've written! I believe I'll publish it someday.

Sometimes we buy or rent a movie. Watching films at home provides us with privacy, new ideas, and techniques to try. Endless movie titles offer both education and entertainment, depending on your interests.

Staff at the stores (or reviews available online) offer guidance to make sure a film provides the desired information. Sometimes I watch the movie alone, sometimes with Steve. I make sure whatever I watch honors and respects women—qualities essential for me in any film I view.

Six months after Steve's surgery, I bought a DVD that taught me how to perform a striptease. As I searched for ways to increase Steve's interest in sex, I thought perhaps if I learned a few sexy dance movements, it would spark his desire. We watched the DVD together, and I became intrigued with the possibility of buying sexy clothes and shoes.

Then, as often happened, Steve didn't exhibit much interest, so I allowed myself to get distracted and discouraged. Once again, I chose to ignore our non-existent sex life and just live with the situation. Given his lack of interest, I didn't want to risk performing a striptease. So I appeased myself with the thought that at least Steve lives cancer free, that he didn't die. I should feel grateful that at least I still have a husband.

As I reflect on this time, I realize I brought my creative *feminine* quality to our relationship by buying this DVD and watching it with Steve. However, I didn't bring my *masculine* quality of implementation to the fore. Thus, nothing happened, and our relationship continued to flounder.

Make Your Choices!

Glance back through this section and review the variety of choices you might take to enhance your sex life after prostate cancer. Determine what activity your body finds most attractive, then use your head to make it happen.

Take action now and face the issues that prevent you from living a thriving life. Avoiding the issues you identify will only delay your happiness, as it did mine.

Planning for Intimacy with a Tantrika

In 2010, three years after Steve's treatment, it became time (once again) to tackle changing our mediocre sex life. I felt concerned that the intimate time Steve and I spent together seemed to go up and down like a roller coaster. Most of the time, we were either going downhill or remaining on a flat track. We continued to live like roommates, not lovers. Compatible roommates, but still, roommates. Naturally, I wanted more in my marriage than a companion; I wanted a partner and a lover.

During an appointment with my naturopath (who helps me stay healthy as I move closer to menopause), she asked about my interest in sex and about Steve's recovery. When I stated we could do much better, she gave me the card for someone who calls herself a Tantrika. Reviewing the Tantrika's website, I learned that a Tantrika lives a life that honors the beauty and fullness of sexuality, using her knowledge to assist others. I set up a series of appointments with her. In fact, Steve and I each met with her alone and as a couple. She asked us a lot of questions, and we asked her a lot of questions. She then presented a number of options to use Tantra to assist us in improving our life together.

One my early dialogues with the Tantrika went something like this:

"Are you feeling any attraction toward Steve?"

"No, not really. I want to be turned on by him, but it's not working now."

"Were you ever attracted to Steve?"

"Yes, sparks flew early in our relationship. We spent a weekend in Sedona learning conscious loving techniques. Our interest in practicing these new skills went away pretty quickly. I'm not sure why. Steve didn't seem very interested, and I became busy with other things."

"Are you very present when you're with him now?"

"Actually, not really. Usually my mind is elsewhere. We don't seem to have much to talk about, and my 'to do' list is really long right now. I'm pretty distracted by other things."

"Do you know the term Beginner's Mind?"

"I read a book that described Beginner's Mind as looking at something with new eyes. It's using curiosity and appreciation, without any preconception. Is that what you mean?"

"Yes. Is that something you'd be willing to try with Steve?"

"I suppose so. I want to look at all of life with a Beginner's Mind. Focusing on that to improve my relationship with Steve is a valuable idea."

"Can you see how bringing a Beginner's Mind to your time with Steve would help you stay more present with him?"

"Yes. I can see how it would force me to be more observant and more awake to what we are experiencing. Thank you. I'll make a point of practicing these techniques."

I spent more time with the Tantrika and reviewed my notes from the conscious loving weekend. As I looked for information on the Internet, I discovered the practice of Tantra began thousands of years ago in Eastern cultures as a spiritual path that includes sensuality and sexuality in its teachings. In the West, many people view Tantra as a practice for experiencing extended orgasms. While some Tantric practices can help extend orgasms, they represent only one aspect of the teachings. Over time, Tantra has become an accumulation of practices and ideas.

For me, Tantra teaches love, presence, and compassion. It also encourages me to focus on energy movement in my body, including sexual energy, and to value the many different aspects of sensuality in my life. It teaches me a healthy view of sexuality and that orgasm need not happen at all to experience a loving connection.

Steve and I continue learning from the Tantrika, who studied with the master known as Osho. She uses her intuition and knowledge to guide her teachings. I doubt if our resistance to some of her suggestions is unusual, but over time, I saw how she provided information essential to our growth as individuals and as a couple.

Part of our conversation with the Tantrika during our first session went like this:

"How much intimate time do you spend with each other now?"

"We shower together every morning and cuddle together before we sleep—that is, when Steve is in town. We also talk some during the day. We're usually pretty busy doing projects on the weekend."

"Would you be willing to spend four hours of uninterrupted time together each week?"

"How much? Four hours? Not a chance. I don't see how I could fit that in. Work is really busy right now, and we just have a lot going on right now."

"What about just two hours a week to enjoy your relationship and explore your physical bodies?" she said with a chuckle, obviously wondering what else in our lives could possibly warrant more importance.

"Cindie, you can find two hours, can't you?"

"Well, I suppose so. Let me look at my calendar when we get home and we can get it scheduled."

"I want you both to commit to this time together no matter what. Even if you just had a fight, feel too busy, or just aren't interested, will you make sure you take the time to 'just do it?'"

"Yes," we both agreed, not realizing how difficult that commitment would be to keep.

At first, it seemed as if everything that could go wrong did. A big work project came up for me the first week, and I asked Steve if we could postpone our session until the next week. The next week came, and we started fighting about something the night before our scheduled session. Neither of us felt like spending time together, much less intimate time. So we didn't.

The Tantrika still pressured us to hold the sessions no matter what was happening in our lives. Noting the importance of this commitment to our relationship, Steve continued to encourage me to make this time a priority. If we truly wanted to become closer, we must invest the time. A new twist, he was taking the masculine role and initiating intimate time together. He was learning new techniques from the Tantrika and saw the possibility of a good sex life. Suddenly our roles reversed. He took the lead, pushing me into intimacy. So although I had initiated the sessions with the Tantrika, for some unknown reason, I became reluctant to spend this time with Steve.

With Steve's insistence, we booked our two-hour intimacy sessions together on a weekly basis. Before long, I opened up to the pleasure and joy that scheduled time brought me. While spontaneity can add excitement to life, I eventually became realistic. Life happens. Sex easily and repeatedly gets postponed and often ignored.

Yet, even with my schedule full of appointments today, I wonder what can possibly be more important than making sure I spend quality, intimate time with my husband.

When Intimacy Isn't a Priority

Looking back, I'm fascinated to see how little time I actually spent engaged with Steve in an intimate way in the past. Yes, it's highly possible a majority of people don't spend much time engaged in intimacy with themselves or with their partners.

As an example, during a group tour vacation, we noticed how little time most couples spent alone together. They got up to watch the birds before the sun rose and then toured all morning. During the free hour after lunch, a few couples spent their time outside writing, looking at photos or talking with others. The afternoon included more tours, dinner, and conversation. Several couples went to bed late each night, got up to watch the birds early the next morning, and repeated this same schedule for the entire 10 days of the tour.

During this trip, Steve and I found it easy to get caught up in the "doing" and not carving out any "being" time. Once we realized this pattern, we made a point of spending our afternoon siesta time alone together, focusing on each other. We talked about forgoing some of the activities to spend time on our relationship—a new concept for me. We also made a point of leaving the dinner conversation early some nights so we could have extra time, just the two of us.

Because we now look at sex differently than we did, we view our vacations differently as well. We *always* plan intimate time together. And because we've committed to making our relationship a priority—creating intimacy in all areas of life—we walk our talk (well, most of the time).

I'm not judging the couples on our trip who spent all their time doing activities and little time alone with each other. We all establish priorities in our lives, either consciously or unconsciously. On previous trips, I didn't *plan* to participate in all the activities; it just happened. Likewise, I never consciously decided to make intimate time with Steve a priority, but that *didn't* happen. After all, we often spent a lot of money to travel on a trip and wanted to "get our money's worth."

But today, given my intention to live a life that thrives, I *require* intimate time with Steve, and with myself, even when we're visiting exotic places.

Talk About Sex a Lot More

Our society doesn't encourage talking about sex with others, but I believe we can improve our world if we talk more about love and sex. I look for opportunities to share with people, in the right way, that Steve and I take time for intimacy so we can experience greater feelings of closeness. I discuss content with others when we read books or take classes about sex. Although I don't offer intimate details, I'm open to answering their questions about sexuality.

By way of example, I also make a point to tell others how much time Steve and I spend on our relationship. When more people open up about sex and share that they make their relationship a priority, it often encourages others to do the same. I suggest even using the topic of prostate cancer to share with friends all the improvements in their sex life.

Open Up Your Creativity

I invite you to share (as you deem appropriate) how you're finding new ways to explore sensuality and sex. Tell others how your prostate cancer experience allowed you to open up your creativity and add more variety than ever before.

Consider revealing how you switch between feminine and masculine roles in your physical relationship. Mention the feedback technique you commonly use with your man. Doing so encourages other women to improve their communication skills.

When you share how you make sex a priority in your relationship, others pick up on your example. It might just lead to creating similar scenes like the one in the film *When Harry Meets Sally*. Remember when Sally fakes an orgasm while she and Harry are lunching? After Sally's orgasmic noises subside, a woman at a nearby table says to the server, "I'll have what she's having."

While you don't have to fake an orgasm in public to talk about sex, why not amp up the time you spend sharing ideas about sex with friends?

Applying Tantric Techniques

The Tantrika continued, using her intuition to guide her to make suggestions that would increase our feelings of intimacy. Although some of her suggestions met with initial resistance, we found them gratifying and healing when we let go and just did them. I share two examples here—bouncing meditation and massage.

Bouncing Meditation

During one of our couples' sessions, the Tantrika asked us to participate in a bouncing meditation. She played a meditation from her teacher, Osho, called the Kundalini Meditation. We started moving up and down in one place, feeling the beat, eyes closed, allowing the energy to spread throughout our bodies. She encouraged us to make any sounds we felt coming up through our bodies, and to just move in whatever way they wanted to go. She said this movement might bring up emotions that we may not be able to explain, but ones we could release to help us heal.

At one point during the bouncing, I wanted to burst into tears. But even though I felt safe and the Tantrika encouraged releasing our emotions, I didn't let go. I stuffed my emotions back into my body, not granting myself the relief that would have accelerated my recovery process.

Fully Release What You're Feeling

I don't like admitting that I had denied myself a chance to heal during this time with the Tantrika. I hope you learn from me and fully release anything you feel in your body. Cry, yell, dance, throw ice cubes. Find ways to experience and release your deepest emotions, no matter what they are or where they came from.

Steve and I frequently bounce to Osho's Kundalini Meditation CD as part of our intimacy sessions. It helps both healthy and unhealthy energy flow through our bodies while dissipating "stuck" energy. I feel more alive after bouncing—more present and more engaged with Steve.

To allow energy to flow through Steve's penis, the Tantrika asked him to use the pump he bought soon after his surgery. She encouraged him to use this vacuum therapy system on a daily basis to get blood and feeling back into his penis, and he believes it makes a difference. Sometimes I assist him, allowing this practice to enhance our intimate time together.

Massage

During our first session with the Tantrika, she insisted we buy a massage table and massage each other on a regular basis. Frankly, we couldn't imagine doing that. After all, we aren't trained massage therapists and didn't want to spend that kind of time rubbing each other. Nor could we imagine investing in a massage table. In our small house, where could we possibly store a bulky massage table? And where would we find one to buy anyway? Used or new? I'm sure the Tantrika thought our excuses and procrastination would never end.

Eventually, we broke down and bought a gently used massage table found through Craigslist. We store it in our closet and get it out almost every weekend—all the time wondering why we waited so long to bring it into our lives!

The Tantrika taught us the importance of healing touch with massage while emphasizing that these sessions didn't need to result in orgasms. Our conversations went something like:

"It seems like you both live in your heads quite a bit with the work you do. Using the massage table will allow you time to focus on your body, really learning to feel it."

An Investment in Intimacy

As you move from just surviving prostate cancer to thriving, learn from our lesson—skip the excuses and save time. Buy a massage table for you and your man. Use it on a weekly basis. Invest in creamy lotion that smells luscious, make sure your house is warm, and stay present as you begin to give and receive pleasure.

"You're right. We both spend a lot of time on the computer every day."

"This time is for you to learn what it's like to listen to your own body, in addition to the other person's body. You can do this most easily through what I call a healing touch. By focusing on helping each other heal, I want you to eliminate any intention that these sessions are about orgasms."

"So what you're saying is this isn't about sex in the traditional sense. This isn't necessarily a massage of the genitals, with an end goal of orgasm?"

"That's correct, Cindie. I want you to take time to connect in a new way, a very intimate way, and without working toward a goal. This time is dedicated to taking care of each other by simply giving and receiving love. You may find that an orgasm occurs because you aren't focusing on it and because you are so in tune with your bodies. Remember, though, reaching orgasm is not your objective. I want you to listen to *your* body and your partner's body during these sessions."

Her advice that we not focus on orgasms took off the pressure. We were relieved to know that neither of us would need to perform or feel disappointed if an orgasm didn't result from our touching. From there, we began to look forward to our intimacy sessions—just taking care of each other.

Typically, we don't systematically alternate sessions between us—that is, I don't expect Steve to massage me this week because I massaged him last week. Each time, we determine which one of us needs special care. Sometimes we plan our sessions and other times we allow them to simply unfold. Some weeks only one of us receives a massage; other weeks we both do.

After our massage or on other days, we extend our joy and healing touch by showering or bathing together. Using a variety of bath products and loofah sponges, we wash each other's bodies and hair. We smell the different aromas, the textures of the scrubs and gels, and especially the opportunity to spend time with each other soaking in warm water.

In the past, I had received regular massage therapy but Steve hadn't. Once we started using our massage table, we were surprised to discover that he enjoyed being touched a lot. He opened up to receiving my gift of simply touching him without any expectation of sexual performance.

For me, massaging Steve allowed me to develop even more compassion—a feminine quality I was nurturing. I discovered that Steve was starved for this type of non-sexual touch. As I realized how much touch meant to him, I appreciated my ability to help him heal in this way.

I also found that massaging Steve gave me the opportunity to get to know his body differently. As the Tantrika instructed, I allowed myself to look at him in a non-sexual way. By expanding my awareness, a new dimension emerged for me in our relationship.

> ### The Gift of Human Touch
>
> Try a variety of nonsexual healing touches with your partner to see what happens in your relationship. If you're not in an intimate relationship with your man, consider giving him a gift certificate for a massage, or offer to provide some nonsexual healing touch for him. You could simply rub his shoulders or his feet, something to help him relax and feel the gift of human touch.

To further connect with each other, I started implementing something from the Tantric-based conscious loving class that Steve and I had taken a few months before we married. Even though we hadn't incorporated all we learned into our lives, this class provided us with a notebook full of ideas that we could use now that we had a greater interest. I had to make sure I didn't beat myself up because we hadn't acted on them earlier. It's important to realize that *timing is everything*—and nine years ago, it simply wasn't the right time for us.

In class, the instructors encouraged us to allow the woman time to get into her body, as it is often more difficult for the woman to become sexually aroused. I started asking Steve to provide me with time alone to prepare for our intimacy session or to just get in touch with myself. It was wonderful to take time just for me—to nurture my femininity and help me become more present in my body.

Discovering Sensuality by Using All Five Senses

Typically, in my time alone, I discover a new world by exploring my five senses. Too often, I find myself running through life, not experiencing as much as I could. What has changed? Now I seek opportunities to engage my senses, especially touch and smell, the ones I tend to ignore more frequently than the others.

This way of living allows me to learn more about my body and helps me stay present. More than that, I realize just about *everything* can become more sensual when I focus on the sensations of my physical body. Activities as mundane as doing the dishes, driving to work, and brushing my teeth acquire new meaning when I experience them in a sensual way.

Recently, I had lunch with a busy woman who said she hardly ever shaves her legs any more, much less takes time to put lotion on her body. She told me she had taken a bath the previous weekend and how refreshing it felt. I invited her to move into the realm of sensuality by including some type of activity each day that involves all five senses. We laughed as she struggled to think of them all: hearing, sight, smell, taste, and touch. She commented that she lives in her head so much, she often forgets about the pleasures of smells and what it's like to eat a meal slowly, tasting every bite.

We talked about focusing on one single sense a day or one sense a week and she selected the sense of smell immediately. Just then our Italian food arrived, giving both of us ample opportunity to savor the delicious aromas of marinara sauce and garlic.

I've read about the value of aromatherapy—using various fragrant essential oils for well-being—and how smells can remind us of pleasant (and unpleasant) times. Unfortunately, ever since I had surgery to clear an infection in my sinus area, my sense of smell has remained weak. As a result, I work extra hard to bring scents into my life. Eucalyptus causes me to think of a spa and all the relaxing pleasures I receive during spa treatments, so I buy eucalyptus room freshener. I learned that the scent Ylang Ylang increases passion for many people, so I bought candles with that fragrance to use during intimacy sessions with Steve. Aromatherapy products such as sprays, diffusers, and incense create mood shifts that I relish. And flowers bring much joy to our home, both in scent and sight.

Scents and Sensuality

Buy a number of different fragrances in candles, incense, and oils for intimacy sessions with your man and discover what memories the scents bring up for each of you. Make it a game to find out if peppermint massage oil really stimulates his body. Let him use lavender-scented lotion on you to see if it relaxes you, as it does many people. If the scent of cookie dough reminds you of your childhood, keep that fragrance out of the bedroom. Experiment to find what scents appeal the most!

My busy lunch companion told me she often eats in her car or snacks while she works. She's not alone; many women eat when they feel stressed. Often, they eat unconsciously, not tasting or enjoying the food. Frequently, they end up eating more than their bodies require, causing possible weight gain. Others lose weight during times of stress. Preoccupied with worry, they don't enjoy the process of eating and don't eat much at all.

Food and Sensuality

You may be one who enjoys cooking and/or eating and finds that food provides you with plenty of sensual opportunities. Regardless of how you currently experience taste, consider how you might incorporate this sense into your intimacy sessions.

Experiment with different foods that seem sensual to you. Make part of your intimacy session an outing to the grocery store, either with your man or by yourself. Set up a game to find sensual foods that appeal to your various senses. Some of my sensual favorites are ripe mangos, figs, chocolate, hot tea, and whipped cream (yes, I call whipped cream a food).

Learning to look at sex in a whole new way can involve creating a buffet of different menu options. I love to spice up my life by adding different tastes.

When I bring the buffet concept into my sense of hearing, Steve's noises come to mind. Whether he purposely makes a noise to make me smile or uses it to release an emotion doesn't matter. I enjoy the sounds because they allow me to connect with him in a special way, and they definitely bring me into the present moment.

Sounds and Sensuality

Like a little boy, your man might overuse a noise that he believes amuses you. Typically, if a man finds something that makes you happy, he won't make a change. After all, if he's getting positive results, he's winning. Why would he take a risk that might cause him to lose by doing something new?

Rather than get angry and complain, let him know you value his noises and would love it if he'd find some *new* ones to share with you. Consider using the request method described earlier by telling him what you want, not what you don't want. The conversation might go like this:

"Steve, can I interrupt? I want to find time to talk with you about something I thought about recently. There's nothing wrong and it's not urgent."

"Can it wait until tomorrow, Cindie? I'm really pushed with this deadline. Will you remind me?"

"Yes, that will be fine and I'll bring it up tomorrow."

"Thanks for taking time to talk about something important to me. I love hearing the noises you make, and it would make me even happier if you surprised me with some new noises. Would you be willing to do that for me?"

"Yes, but what if you don't like my new noises?"

"I doubt if that will happen, Steve. If it happens, I'll let you know, though. Is there anything I can do to support you in creating a variety of noises?"

"If you make new noises to give me some ideas, I'm willing to give this a try."

"Thank you, Steve. Your new noises will help me feel even happier. Grrrr. How's that for a new noise?"

"I like it, Cindie. I'll see what I can do."

My noises bring a lot of feedback into my relationship with Steve. By making various sounds, I let him know when to continue or stop what he's doing. Especially during massage or sex, my sounds can guide him to pleasing me more or moving to a different spot. My personal favorite sounds are mmm, oh, and ham, pronounced haahhmmnng—or a combination of these.

Music offers an obvious way to increase awareness of our sense of hearing, and it can help create the desired ambiance. For example, as my friend and I finished our meal at the Italian restaurant, we tuned into the music playing in the background, agreeing that it transported us to Italy. I feel fortunate to live in a world where technology offers a huge variety of sounds and easy access to music that fits all kinds of moods.

Music and Sensuality

Consider compiling a special music playlist for intimate times with your man or to begin your intimacy sessions. Create a playlist together or plan ahead and surprise each other with new ones.

Back at the restaurant, I asked my friend if she would consider taking just three minutes each morning to give herself a dry massage or a massage with oil. Health experts write about the benefits of making sure our bodies get touched all over every day, and not a lot of time is needed.

Briskly running our hands over areas of the body before showering provides a perfect way to detoxify the body's tissues, increase circulation, and enhance the immune system, according to The Chopra Center. Adding oil can provide a pleasant aroma to the experience. It will also keep your skin soft and allow your hands to move more sensually over your body. Called an Abhyanga, or self-abhy, this ritual is part of the practice of the ancient science of life called Ayurveda.

(Find out more about this type of massage at *www.chopra.com/abhy*.) Doing this before my morning shower launches my day with vitality.

Awareness of my senses can occur in surprising ways. Something as routine as getting dressed in the morning provides me the opportunity to focus on touch. I experience the different textures of fabrics—the smooth feel of silk and the softness of cotton. My desire to enjoy this sense requires that I remain present when I get dressed rather than stay in my head planning my day.

As I become more aware of the fabrics that touch my body, I find that my sensitivity to all touch increases. Now, when Steve touches me, I'm much more aware of his touch and feel it more intensely. This gives me immense pleasure and Steve another opportunity to "win."

Most people use the sense of sight more frequently than the others. I shared with my friend that creating an environment of beauty all around me—beautifying my home, yard, and office—helped to enhance my life after prostate cancer.

If I'm not present, I just don't see some of the art in our home; I rush by it every day. In my hurry, I used to pull out the same drinking glass every day. Becoming more aware of this habit caused me to find glasses in the back cupboard that I enjoy using selectively.

As my friend and I walked out of the restaurant, we stood together for a moment, listening to the birds and the traffic, and feeling the sun on our skin. We spent an extra minute hugging each other, breathing together to bring ourselves completely into our bodies. I then spent the rest of the day more present than usual—and I suspect she did too!

Environment of Joy

After the traumatic experience of cancer, I encourage you to make changes in your home by moving artwork, replacing dishes, or recovering furniture. These projects tap into your feminine qualities to create an environment that brings you joy everywhere you look.

If, like me, you find doing projects around the house too stressful, then hire the right kind of help to make sure you create beauty in your surroundings. Invite a friend to help or hire someone who can look through your eyes to assist you in finding just the right items that bring you pleasure. Sit in each room, gaze around to determine what annoys you, and then replace those items as soon as you can.

If your spaces already provide the right environment for you, spend time enjoying the views and practicing being in the moment.

Moving Energy to Achieve Orgasm

For many couples, sex mostly revolves around intercourse and orgasm. That's what Steve and I experienced in the beginning of our relationship. Then, within our first six months together, we attended a conscious loving class for two-and-a-half (long) days. There, we learned how to look at sex in an entirely different way. The techniques we practiced were designed to please each other sexually and they helped us bond after our prostate cancer journey. Overall, the class opened our eyes about how to use energy to experience orgasms. For example, did you know that energy can be used to create an orgasm in a man without ejaculation, often called a dry orgasm? That intrigued me.

New Way to Look at Sex and Orgasm

The instructors taught us that a man can learn to delay his ejaculation to provide more pleasure to the woman. This extends the opportunity for her to achieve orgasm and enhances his own pleasure. The man can then join the woman in her orgasms by moving his energy with hers, allowing the couple to experience hours of pleasure. Admittedly, this concept was difficult for me to understand and foreign to what I'd ever experienced. My knowledge about sex had started out, and remained, traditional. However, this conscious loving information gave us a different way to look at sex.

During this class, Steve and I discovered how men could slow down, view sex as more than intercourse, and enjoy intimate time with their partner without the goal of reaching an orgasm. As a result, we began to look at our lovemaking as a journey, not a destination for orgasm. When we returned home, we practiced these new techniques diligently—at least at first. We brought the concept of "five minutes a day" into our lives to help us connect by spending at least five minutes each day in an intimate way. Because we were gradually discovering more about ourselves, we were happy to dedicate time to practicing what we'd learned.

As with many things that bring growth to one's life, however, discomfort arose. We started to feel afraid of the vulnerability of allowing someone "in" so close. After a while, the rewards didn't come fast enough for us, and we bumped up against our own fears. Slowly, we lost interest in this new way of looking at sex. Our intimacy languished.

As mentioned earlier, when we started spending time with the Tantrika in 2010, we drew upon our knowledge from the conscious loving class we'd taken almost a decade before. Little did we know at the time that it was laying the foundation we would later need so desperately for looking at sex in a whole different way.

Still, this new perspective wasn't what Steve wanted. Instead, he wanted his old sex life back—that comfortable feeling of intercourse and orgasm. He wanted to ejaculate to reach the goal. He wanted to "win."

Once we started talking about it, I discovered that my memory of our sex life before prostate cancer differed significantly from Steve's. For me, his recollection of our sex life seemed more like what he probably experienced in college and in his 20s. However, he clearly wanted our sex life to improve, and he was upset that it wasn't happening. It took time to get Steve to the point of envisioning a sex life that differed from his memories—a sex life that didn't involve the goal of orgasm. This required him to take risks and learn new skills in an area that frightened him. Indeed, we both had to learn how to respond in healthy ways when erection and orgasm weren't always among the options. I had to learn not to take it personally when Steve's body didn't respond. Like anything new, it took time and practice.

Gradually, we redefined our sex life, adding as much humor as possible. Today, we still recognize our vulnerability and encourage each other to experiment. And because we no longer look at orgasm as the endpoint of our intimate time together, we now enjoy more freedom than before.

Honestly, I had wanted a *better* sex life well before Steve's prostate cancer diagnosis, yet my memories brought frustration and disappointment to mind. Why would I want to go back to that? I'm grateful that, due to our renewed commitment and training, our sex life blossomed significantly.

Making Sexual Time Together a Priority

Today, scheduling time for intimacy means we make sex a priority in our lives, not something we do if we have time or because it's our anniversary. It provides us the opportunity to prepare for it all week, increasing our desire for each other and resulting in fireworks for both of us. As we glean new ideas from books and movies, we experience more creativity in bed.

Looking at sex in this new way gives me time to be in my body. The sensitivity of our bodies has increased because we learned to slow down. We've moved our focus from the genitals to paying attention to what feels good in other places. As we experiment with moving energy and using our female and male energies in a balanced way, the sparks fly.

Yes, You *Can* Make Changes

Do you have negative feelings about your past sex life? Perhaps your man wanted intercourse frequently and you didn't enjoy it. Pleased that your man no longer expresses an interest in sex, you may privately celebrate when he experiences difficulty achieving an erection. It may be a relief to you that having sex is no longer "required" as part of your relationship.

If you didn't enjoy traditional sex, know that you *can* make changes. The prostate cancer experience gives you an opportunity to enhance intimacy without the parts you didn't like. Consider the options suggested and select the ones that don't feel threatening to you. As you and your man become closer emotionally, perhaps you'll feel more comfortable adding other components.

If you haven't discovered what sexual fulfillment means to you, what a great time to find out!

I continue using all the techniques described in this section to create even more sexual fulfillment for myself—because a satisfying sex life causes me to thrive.

CHAPTER 3
THRIVING EMOTIONALLY

FOR THE LONGEST TIME, I thought thriving after prostate cancer meant just getting our sex life back. I didn't realize it meant becoming more intimate and vulnerable with Steve, but I now know that moving beyond survival involves more than our physical relationship.

My prostate cancer experience provided a catalyst for me to address other matters in my life that prevented me from feeling happy. I had safely tucked them away, but they required a closer look before I could heal. My journey highlighted wounds from my childhood and emphasized unhealthy patterns in my life. It became clear I didn't want to continue the strained life I had been living.

Reducing Fear by Gaining Knowledge

One of my best teachers has defined fear as simply a lack of knowledge. As I look back over my prostate cancer experience, I can see the fear that ruled me throughout Steve's diagnosis, surgery, and recovery. It also showed up in the form of avoiding intimacy with him. Living with this fear put me straight in survival mode.

I'm guessing you did a much better job than I did to reduce your fears by going to medical appointments with your man and researching answers to your questions. I didn't engage much in Steve's search for the best treatment and recovery approach. However, he seemed to prefer it that way, making it easy for me to make other activities a priority. He answered all my questions as best he could, yet there was still so much we didn't know. And my fears prevailed.

Once I finally decided to gain more knowledge about Steve's recovery, I asked questions before and after his quarterly appointments with his urologist. I found information on the Internet and skimmed a few books to help me understand the experiences of other couples. These resources helped, but they primarily gave me knowledge about Steve's *physical* recovery. I couldn't find much about my own *emotional* recovery and how to improve my life after prostate cancer. The urologist viewed Steve, not me, as his patient—and rightly so. The doctor's job was to remove the cancer in Steve's body, not treat my emotional ups and downs.

Not surprisingly, fears related to Steve's diagnosis and recovery activated other fears in my life, further contributing to my emotional upheaval. I explored first one healing path and then another. I read books, went to conferences, and counseled with a variety of individuals. I gained value from most of these experiences, but no one gave me a road map. In fact, I don't believe one exists for this type of journey—for me or for you. I do believe, though, that you can learn from my experiences to assist in your emotional recovery after prostate cancer.

Learn, Experiment, Share

Consider the healing methods and modalities I used and find something that works for you. Share your experiences with others, and let's collectively learn how to live a life that thrives.

A wealth of offerings is available on the Internet, so be sure to search for the topics you'd like to know more about. Community colleges, libraries, and churches also offer opportunities to learn.

Individual counseling, coaching, and healing sessions may speak to you. If you don't know how you learn best, experiment with a variety of methods. You may prefer individual or group sessions, audio or video programs, books, or classes. Energy work in which you release emotions may be your ticket. Discover the ways you like to obtain information so you can best heal. Consider using your prostate cancer experience to change unhealthy patterns and clear up hurtful childhood issues. When you do, your life will truly thrive.

Healing Through Various Modalities

My mother tells me that my father would have been a better dad if counseling, self-help books, and therapy had been more accepted during his lifetime. He read a lot, valued education, and liked to learn. Back then, though, the personal growth business didn't exist. In fact, people thought those who sought counseling were crazy.

Fortunately, our culture today more readily accepts those who seek assistance with emotional challenges than it did when my dad was living. Many people receive various types of therapy, using a broad range of professionals trained in specific areas.

I enjoy learning about new healing modalities and trying different ones, but I tended at first to move from one healing method to another too quickly. Sometimes I didn't experience the full benefit of a technique because I didn't allow myself enough time to assimilate it into my being. I also looked *outside* myself for answers when many of the necessary answers had to come from *within* me. I admit; I enjoyed the distraction of reading another book, listening to another audio session, or taking a new class.

However, as I became clearer about my goals and identified the major issues I faced, I started hearing my inner voice louder than ever. As I listened to it, I discovered methodologies that worked for me and stayed with them, doing the hard work required rather than moving on to the next healing method on the list.

Look Within Yourself

Identify the patterns in your life that cause you unhappiness and strain your relationship, then allow your inner voice to guide you to healing modalities that will best serve you. Ask experts to assist in identifying what prevents you from living a life that thrives. Then find the right teachers to help you clear away issues that hold you back.

Your most precious guide on your journey to thriving emotionally after prostate cancer is within you. That's why my advice throughout this guide focuses on you, not your man.

How did I emotionally shift my life out of survival mode? Let me describe the most effective methods for me.

Cellular Memory

Over the years, I've read about a concept called cellular memory in which both the body and the brain store emotional information. One way this shows up is when transplant patients start exhibiting characteristics of those whose organ they received. Gary Swartz, Ph.D. and his co-workers at the University of Arizona have documented a number of these intriguing cases.

My reading tells me that unhealthy memories stored in the body cause disease and discomfort. My body stores information that causes me to act in unconscious ways based on past behavior. Today, I work with Sherry Anshara, founder of QuantumPathic® Center of Consciousness *(www.quantumpathic.com)*. Sherry facilitates my healing by assisting me to release the past from my cellular memory where it no longer serves me and guide me to change limiting belief systems.

Sherry developed the QuantumPathic® Energy Method (QPEM) more than 20 years ago using a merger of science and spirituality. She teaches students and clients to understand the patterns and behaviors in their lives. Each QPEM session is unique based on the individual. Through dialogue or dialogue combined with touch/movement, individuals receive their own personal answers to heal their issues.

From working with Sherry, I've learned to respond consciously to situations in my life rather than automatically repeating unhealthy patterns from the past. For example, I've carried around the pattern of relying on the validation of other people for my happiness. As noted earlier, I once looked to Steve to validate me as a woman through his interest in me sexually. When he didn't, or couldn't, provide that validation by saying something like "Cindie, you're really great in my eyes," my happiness meter plummeted.

I finally realized that to become the person I desired, I had to validate *myself*. I'm the only one I can control, and I'm the only one I can change. Conversely, I can't make Steve desire me as a woman, and I can't force him to open up to me.

Here's the good news. By taking classes and investing in private sessions with Sherry, I've eliminated my need to be validated by other people, including Steve. Changing this *one* belief has given me a freedom and power I never even knew existed!

Changing Stories

At a business meeting I attended in January, 2011, the facilitator asked participants to share the most important lesson learned during the last year. After some thought, my answer related to a specific event that had happened six months earlier.

A conversation with a friend caused me to change my story after I mentioned I needed to hear from someone to reach closure with a relationship. "Cindie," she challenged me, "what story are you telling yourself about this situation? How can you need something that depends on another person?" As I looked at her sheepishly, I said, "You're right. I really was telling myself a story that didn't have an ending. Do you have any suggestions to help me reach closure?" As so many great coaches do, she turned the question back to me. "What do *you* think you can do?" She was right. I had my own answer. "It's going to be a combination of meditation, journaling, and sharing my ideas with others to sort through what I've learned and reach peace with this experience," I answered.

A month later, with a lot of contemplation and writing behind me, I let my friend know I'd reached closure with this relationship without hearing from the other person. I had changed my story by looking within and finding exactly what I needed to return to a place of gratefulness, harmony, and love.

All this happened while taking a PAX class (a series of classes described in the next section) with another friend.

One evening during dinner, I shared my journey with her. "I feel really close to putting this experience behind me. Something is still missing, though." As we continued talking, I suddenly burst out, "I've got it! Tonight I'm going to write letters to the person involved, getting it all out of my system. I've used this technique before, and it really works for me." I immediately felt a sense of peace, allowing me to enjoy the rest of the evening with my friend.

Back in my hotel room that night, I drafted three letters. One was from Little Cindie, crying out her disappointment and hurt for what happened. Another was from a grown-up and very angry Cindie who used words that hadn't been uttered in decades. The venom and hostility that came out of my pen caused me to blush. It even frightened me.

The last letter I wrote was also from a grown-up Cindie. This letter, though, came from a calm, conscious, and loving Cindie. In it, I reflected on what the experience had provided me. I thanked the person for participating in a moment that allowed me to break a pattern in my life—one I didn't want to repeat. I apologized for my behavior and asked for forgiveness.

I didn't sleep as well as I anticipated that night. When I woke up in the morning, something seemed to be missing. After my meditation and shower, another flash came to me. To reach complete closure, I required a letter written *by* Cindie *to* Cindie. I quickly sat at the desk and wrote a letter to myself. In it, I congratulated Cindie on growing so much and breaking the pattern, reminding her that she didn't require another person to validate her. I signed the letter "I love you, Cindie," put my pen down, and felt a beautiful stillness.

I wasn't finished yet. I took all four letters into the bathroom. Through my tears and runny nose, I read each letter out loud to myself. Then I tore up each one and flushed all four down the toilet. With that last flush, I felt all the hurt, pain, anger, and disappointment disappear from my body, leaving me with what I sought—complete appreciation and love for the individual and the moment itself. I had moved forward in a positive way. I had accepted not being able to control what someone else does or doesn't do. Clearly, I was able to change my story based on what I could control.

In fact, I was able to change *a lot* of my stories by participating in The Sedona Intensive. (I described this program and my male dark side, Charlie, in Chapter 2.) After I read Albert Gaulden's book, *You're Not Who You Think You Are*, Steve and I participated in The Sedona Intensive both as individuals and as a couple. This weeklong program challenged me more than anything else in my life. I learned even more than I had before about my limiting beliefs and how to eliminate them. In the process, the unconscious roles I played became visible, allowing true transformation to occur.

Toward the end of the program, I had an encounter with Albert that he called "transference." As mentioned earlier, I don't fully understand psychological terminology, but here's what happened. During my morning session with Albert, in a loud voice, I burst out, "Albert, you aren't listening to me. I'm talking, and you're not hearing me. I'm scared of you, and I can't even look at you." I was shaking in my seat, tears pouring down my cheeks so much, I could barely see Albert's big smile. "That's what you needed to do, Cindie," he assured me. "You found the courage to speak your truth, *transferring* your childhood pain of not being heard by men onto me."

The Sedona Intensive resulted in a number of similar break-throughs for me, forcing me to look at all aspects of my life in detail. It required me to clear issues with my parents, with past relationships, with Steve, and with myself. During that time, I wrote about my anger, my sadness, my disappointment, and my fears. I wrote until my fingers couldn't hold a pen any longer.

In the process, chiropractic treatments helped me release old traumas or stories. A hypnotherapist helped me examine my relationships with my mom and dad in other ways. I forgave my dad for many things, saw him through new eyes, and con-nected with him differently, even though he had died years ago. With the help of a psychologist, I finally saw and understood the destructive patterns in my intimate relationships. I learned about something called *triangulation* that had haunted me throughout the decades. This knowledge allowed me to work through an encounter with another man that had the potential to end my relationship with Steve.

Once I understood my behaviors, I found ways to change my patterns—and happily stay in my marriage. I accepted the fact that I couldn't change Steve, and that he may or may not change on his own. I knew no one could improve my life but me. I took complete responsibility for healing my wounds from the past and let go of harmful patterns.

What Healing Modalities Work for You?

Whether or not you enjoyed a perfect childhood, if you're strug-gling after surviving prostate cancer, explore a healing modality that appeals to you. For me, a combination of traditional and non-traditional methods made a huge difference.

To summarize, clearing these emotional traumas allowed me to release the past emotional "hooks"—and thrive in the present.

Learning about Men

Much of my ability to thrive after prostate cancer has depended on how well I could relate to the man in my life. As I learned more about the differences between men and women, I found ways to understand men overall—to accept our differences and communicate with them to get my needs met.

Thankfully, about six months after Steve's prostate cancer surgery, I discovered PAX Programs, co-founded by Alison Armstrong and Joan McClain. PAX offers excellent material for women to learn about men and to learn about themselves. (See Resources section for more details.) The title of the first course I took sums up my experience eloquently: "Celebrate Men, Satisfy Women."

What a concept! Although I thought celebrating men was an interesting idea, I really wanted to learn how to satisfy women. After all, Steve didn't meet my needs; I was motivated to find ways to reach him and get my satisfaction back. And if I learned how to celebrate Steve and other men along the way, great!

After attending the first class, I immediately looked at men differently. I began appreciating them for what they bring to the world and looking at life through their eyes. As I did this, I saw Steve—and his response to his prostate cancer—in a new light. I understood that men take care of their own needs first. They don't regard this as selfish; rather, they see it as a necessity in order for them to do anything else in life. No wonder I felt like I couldn't reach Steve after his diagnosis! I came to realize that his entire being was focused on getting healthy so he could have a relationship with me *after* he became cancer free.

I confirmed this understanding several times after class through audio programs and e-books from various authors, learned more about how men think and, more important, how I could better relate to them. A priority was improving my relationship with all the men in my life: Steve, his son, men in the workplace and where I volunteer, and any other man I encounter. Numerous times I listened to the program, "What Husbands Can't Resist" by Bob Grant, L.P.C. It helped me understand why and how I could yield to a man from a position of strength.

While I thought I knew a lot from living and working with men my entire life, I discovered that much of my knowledge served only to *destroy* relationships rather than value our differences. I learned that my quest for independence and my determination not to rely on men actually *inhibited* powerful partnerships.

Steve liked the "new me" so much that he kept encouraging me to attend PAX classes and read more on the topic. He appreciated the communication technique I began using (the one I model throughout this book). He valued how I waited for him to think before he spoke, allowing him to fully gather his thoughts. He felt more respected by me and observed that I'd become happier in our marriage than before.

With his blessing, I attended the PAX course "Celebrate Women" and took further courses called "Men and Sex" and "Men and Marriage." I also read material from other experts—all with the goal to improve my skills so my life would thrive after prostate cancer.

PAX also offers a class for men called "Understanding Women." When Steve and I attended this class together, I found myself in tears several times after identifying with information that I hadn't been able to communicate. As a result, Steve and I now share a common language that assists us when we disagree or are triggered by something in the past.

During this time, Steve read David Deida's *The Way of the Superior Man*. Deida's material instigated hours of conversation. Steve told me he learned how a man can thrive in a world that doesn't look like it did years ago and took in information about women that immediately improved our relationship. For example, in Chapter 17, Deida encourages men to praise women, stating, "The masculine grows by challenge, but the feminine grows by praise." That made quite an impression. After that, Steve increased his compliments of how I looked, showed appreciation for my contributions to our relationship, and gave specific examples of how he saw me succeeding at work.

With our sex life improving and Steve feeling less masculine than before his prostate cancer treatment, he found it crucial to reinforce traits that caused him to feel masculine. For one, he relearned the importance of making decisions. By talking about it, I came to understand the value this masculine trait brought to his healing process.

In fact, as our communication skills improved, Steve became comfortable with my not following his recommendation at certain times, thus appreciating that feminine quality in me. (While I call that feminine quality "freedom to change my mind," others might use less flattering words like "rebellious" or "stubborn.")

I also learned to defer to his expertise more often, knowing that helped him feel more masculine. For example, if I asked him which shoes looked better with an outfit, in the past he might not have answered me because I didn't always follow his recommendations. That threatened his masculine authority. After reading Deida's book, though, Steve was more inclined to decisively give me his answer *and* accept that I might not do what he suggested.

As I became more aware of the importance of decision-making to Steve's masculinity, I found it easier to defer to his preferences. In the past, I would insist on getting my way, something I was used to in business interactions. These days, Steve chooses what meal we take out of the freezer when I ask for his preference—*and* I make sure if I ask this question, I don't care what we eat. In the past, I would ask and then not accept his answer because I wanted something else, but I now know that doesn't help Steve's healing process. Plus it was an unhealthy pattern I needed to break. While decisions around clothing and meals seem mundane, they have provided me with easy ways to change my behaviors—and experience a joyful difference in how I live.

Differing Communication Styles

Steve and I discovered that our various teachers agree with each other in most areas. By studying a variety of material, we hear the same message communicated in different ways using different stories. Yes, we have found some contradictions, *and* we value the opportunity to process our understanding of what the experts say. This lets us verify which messages ring true for us.

One area many experts agree on is learning how to listen to men. In general, women talk more than men because we tend to find verbal communication easy and natural. Not so with most men—and not so with Steve. He prefers to contemplate awhile before he responds. I used to think he was ignoring me or didn't want to talk about the subject, but no more.

Still, I find it difficult to give Steve the time he needs to verbalize a thought and especially to verbalize a feeling. My impatience kicks in, and I want to move on to the next subject. Then I get upset because he doesn't answer me quickly.

Now I know that many men operate like Steve; they need more time to get their words out. If I can keep my mouth shut, I often get responses to the questions I pose. While I wait, I practice deep breathing. It helps me stay present, not get distracted, and not move on to another topic before Steve finishes talking about the first one.

I also use statements that aim at clarification and open-ended questions to help him further develop what he wants to communicate. They might be stated like this: "Tell me more," "Can you clarify that?" "What does that mean?" and "Is there anything else?" Such prompting can keep the conversation going for quite a while. Steve finds these questions most valuable when we talk about intimate topics that involve feelings.

Many times, I don't understand the point Steve is making, so asking an open-ended question allows me to gather more information. It also prevents me from judging Steve and shutting down the conversation. In the past, I'd get angry at him for not answering a question or not talking with me. I didn't realize he didn't believe he had enough chance to respond. The angrier I became, the more he withdrew. The more withdrawn he became, the angrier I'd get. Before long, we found ourselves in a downward spiral faced with a situation that doesn't allow for a constructive resolution of any problem.

During a hike with a girlfriend, I asked if I could dump my frustrations on her about Steve not talking with me at breakfast. "Would you be willing to listen to me about something Steve's doing that really bugs me?" Not knowing what she was in for, she agreed. "He just sits at the table during breakfast, looking at his cereal, shoveling it in his mouth, and eating in complete silence. If I want any conversation to occur, *I* have to initiate it," I whined. "If he's not interested in talking, I'd rather read a magazine than just sit there in silence. And you know how my schedule has been lately," I continued my complaining. "I'm in so many meetings during the day and then all those dinner meetings . . . we hardly have a chance to talk *except* at breakfast."

My anger dissipated after my tirade. That's when I realized I was making a lot of assumptions about his behavior. I confessed that I told Steve I didn't think he cared about me because he ignores me during breakfast. My friend listened and asked, "Do you know why Steve doesn't talk much during breakfast?" I couldn't answer that because I had never asked. Plus, I hadn't given him the space to talk the other morning when I blew up. He had clearly withdrawn because of my anger. So I resolved to talk with him the next day, and the conversation went something like this:

"Steve, I apologize for getting angry the other morning at breakfast. I'd like to start the conversation over, and I'll commit not to get angry. Would you be willing to talk now?"

"Yes. What do I do if you get angry again, though?"

"You can remind me of my commitment, and perhaps I can take a break from the conversation. As I mentioned the other day, I like to talk with you at breakfast, as it helps me connect with you. Sometimes it seems like you're far away, lost in your own thoughts. Am I right?"

"Yes. Often I'm planning my day, so I guess I'm not focused on talking with you. Plus, you wake up more quickly than I do. Sometimes I just don't want to engage in the morning. Can we connect another way, Cindie?"

"I suppose I could learn how to feel connected to you without talking. Perhaps we could establish a ritual before we go our separate ways after breakfast that would allow me to feel close to you. We could try hugging for a longer time and consciously breathing together during the hug. Would that work for you?"

"Yes, I can do that. We can start this morning."

"Great. I believe that will give me the feeling of connection I miss when we don't talk during breakfast. Thank you for working through this with me."

Too often, my venting has harmed Steve's sense of masculinity, as it probably did that morning at breakfast. He reacted as many people do when faced with an angry person; he retreated and didn't engage with me. My unkind words only served to increase his sense of uncertainty about life and himself.

With Steve's sense of who he is as a man possibly in question because of the prostate cancer, learning to better communicate with him allows me to support his recovery. Likewise, supporting his recovery supports my healing, allowing me to thrive.

In addition to listening differently to Steve, I learned how my anger negatively affects him. Venting with my girlfriend provided an outlet for me to release my anger in a safe way that doesn't damage my relationship with Steve.

When I want to vent, I make a point to vent only with a girlfriend who will first listen and then assist me in eventually seeing the situation in a more productive way. I vent for about 10 minutes. Once I'm done, she knows to ask me questions to help me see the situation through Steve's eyes. She doesn't allow me to go back into complaint mode. Instead, she forces me to stay with the process until I can calmly look at the situation through new eyes and empathize with Steve.

After going through this process, I'm in a much better place to use the feedback method when addressing an issue with Steve. Often, I find I don't need to talk with him at all, realizing I misread the situation or I resolved the matter just by venting.

These days, I search for ways to set Steve up to "win" and sense his manhood, his self-confidence. Not all men outwardly show these feelings, and not all men respond in this way. But male or female, we appreciate the opportunity to do something well and receive praise for it. I believe it's important to set our men up to "win" because when they win, we win, too.

Use His Strengths

I enjoy looking for opportunities to use Steve's strengths. For example, he finds it fun to implement better technology for us and does a great job keeping our home equipped with useful tools. Now, I don't get much joy from learning new technology and making sure it works well, and I could easily overlook all that Steve does. However, our technology needs offer a number of opportunities to help him "win." I can let him know how much I appreciate the tools he provides for me to do my work, keep our financial records, and communicate with friends via email. I can show him appreciation when I'm able to quickly find photos on my computer thanks to him, and when he backs up our information on a regular basis.

I know that reinforced behavior typically creates more of the same actions, but the approach has backfired on me, albeit in a humorous way. Steve was jazzed because he purchased a larger computer monitor for me—and he got a great deal on it. He also bought an amazing arm to make it easier for me to adjust its height and thus get rid of the book I had been using to lift up my old monitor. Wow! How exciting! Or so he thought.

Problem: I didn't *want* a bigger monitor and found it difficult to use the larger screen. This situation created more work for me at a very busy time. I struggled to find a way to appreciate his gift, but I found myself getting angry at him. In fact, I blew up at him. "Steve, you know how busy I am and how stressed I'm feeling right now. Didn't you realize that making this kind of change would be hard for me? Don't you ever think about me? I can't get my work done quickly, and everything is in a new place on the monitor. I think you just like big monitors and wanted another one."

As I calmed down and attempted to mop up this situation, I encouraged myself to re-learn this lesson: Vent with a girlfriend first. Once I found myself able to talk with him about this situation, we agreed to new ground rules. He'd talk with me about any changes to technology that he'd like to provide for me. If he can't convince me of their value, the changes won't happen. And if I do want those changes, we'd coordinate their timing, making sure it works for both of us.

Ironically, when a girlfriend visited us one day, she commented on my new monitor the minute she saw it, remarking, "You're so lucky, Cindie, to have that big screen. Don't you just love it?" Steve and I laughed out loud and then shared our story with her.

Faking Appreciation Won't Serve You

Consider complimenting your man only when what he gives you provides value for you. Faking appreciation will not serve you well. While I didn't fake my appreciation for all the technology Steve provided me, he got confused when I didn't appreciate the new monitor.

On the other hand, if your man is so strong in his masculinity that he doesn't balance it well with his feminine qualities, perhaps he could use assistance in this area. For example, you could let him know you support him in showing feelings of sadness and grief with you and might encourage him to release his feelings by crying.

Steve's parents died many years before I met him, but he never fully grieved their loss. Now, each year when we formally remember his mom and dad at the anniversaries of their deaths, I provide an environment where Steve can mourn his loss and cry.

It's helpful to find ways to provide a safe space for our men to show vulnerability and softness. As women, we can observe the feminine qualities they may not embrace, encouraging them to bring them out. Often men can express their feminine qualities through their hobbies, so we can encourage them to nurture a garden, use creativity in woodworking, explore photography, or whatever suits the person best.

Escaping

As we move from surviving toward thriving, it's important to determine whether we escape in healthy or unhealthy ways. Too often, we run away from problems, keeping ourselves so busy that we don't feel the pain. Women tend to escape by taking care of family and/or home, shopping, reading, exercising, surfing the Internet, or spending time with girlfriends. And sometimes we escape by using alcohol or drugs.

Often, we *know* when we're escaping to avoid difficulties in life, when we're spending too much time avoiding the pain of a specific situation. We *know* when we're drinking too much or spending too much money to medicate ourselves.

Let's face it: Escaping in harmful ways keeps us in survival mode. Surviving is a primitive way to live that doesn't allow much joy and passion in our lives. When we just survive, too often we can't fully experience happiness when it arrives because our senses are dulled from covering up the pain for so long.

In the book, *When Things Fall Apart*, Chödrön encourages us to lean into our pain and to really feel it. She says that until we truly feel our pain, we can't get over it. So rather than covering up the pain, no matter where it comes from, we can lean into it, allowing the pain to hurt more than anything we've ever felt. Oddly, this attention will help it to dissipate.

Getting Away

"Escaping" and "getting away" are different experiences. Escaping is usually an unhealthy way of avoiding pain. Alternatively, getting away provides new ideas and perspectives. Time away with girlfriends or daughters plus time alone offer powerful ways to heal. These types of experiences nurture the feminine in us and give us time to reflect with people who listen, share, and empathize.

Spend Time with Thriving Women

Along your journey, make sure you spend time away with the right kind of people. Find women who thrive in their relationships, who move through adversity in healthy ways, and who support you in your healing process. Avoid those individuals who want to complain about their mate, who avoid personal growth, and live with a lot of anger.

Many of my friends find time with their girlfriends to be more valuable than anything else. I'm not one who spends weekends with the girls or who plans spa dates with a group of friends, though. My healing process involves time alone and one-on-one sessions with close friends. I love to travel and get away from my usual routine, with or without a friend. For me, a different environment provides the opportunity to gain new perspectives.

Recently, Steve's son Sean and his girlfriend visited us during their spring break. We spent time in Sedona, a beautiful town two hours north of Phoenix. I decided not to spend the day at the Grand Canyon with them due to some work commitments, but I arranged my schedule so I could hike a new trail into the beautiful red rocks before I drove back to Phoenix. During that hike, I celebrated my decision to spend time alone and at work instead of feeling guilty about not spending the day at the Grand Canyon. In the past, this would not have been possible.

During the hike, I stayed present, enjoying the hawk that flew overhead, marveling at the array of spring colors that appeared around each corner. As I returned, the thought came to me that I still needed to forgive myself for some issues surrounding Steve's prostate cancer diagnosis. I made a commitment to do that the weekend after Sean and his girlfriend returned home.

What's Your Best Getaway?

Determine how you can best get away to find space to heal, laugh, and possibly cry. Try a new experience to help you shift your perspective about a matter. Look at a situation from a different viewpoint. Move yourself toward your own fulfillment—all the way to thriving.

Ironically, when I talked with Steve late that night after they'd returned from the trip to the Grand Canyon, he sounded more alive than I had heard him sound for a while. Despite leaving early and driving for many hours at night, he had high energy and a new outlook on life. While I needed a hike by myself to fulfill me, Steve received a gift by being with people he loves.

Forgiveness

The advantages of practicing forgiveness get a lot of press these days. From our childhoods, parents encourage us to forgive others. Now, we hear more about the importance of forgiving ourselves. This practice is likely to provide relief in the healing process. I know it helped mine.

Whether we write letters and burn them, confess our transgressions to a religious figure, or find other methods of forgiveness, let's make sure we do it—and do it often.

When I went through the Sedona Intensive, I got upset the first day because Albert wanted me to do forgiveness work. I'd done so much work in this area, I didn't think I had anything more to forgive. Albert pushed; I resisted. He pushed some more, and I resisted even harder. Eventually I gave in, accepting that my forgiveness "onion" will probably always have more layers for me to peel. Then, as I began to understand my triangulation pattern, I could see what my dad and other relatives had done to cause me to set men up to fail. Recognizing that, I forgave these individuals for their part in this. I also forgave myself for all the hurt I had caused others because of this unconscious behavior. As I continue to learn and grow, I know I'll uncover more wounds that need healing and more people, including myself, to forgive.

As I discovered on that hike in Sedona, I still took some responsibility for Steve's diagnosis. I thought if I had been a better wife, perhaps he would still have his prostate. Possibly if I had provided better meals or a more loving environment, cancer would not have grown in his body. These thoughts may appear odd. After all, I take responsibility for too many things that don't belong to me, and Steve's cancer is just one of them. So I decided to write a letter of forgiveness to myself, intending to forgive myself. In my journal, I wrote the following:

Dear Cindie,

I forgive you for taking responsibility and beating yourself up over Steve's prostate cancer. You can only take responsibility for your life and your actions. You cannot cause something to happen in another person. Steve remains responsible for his life, his actions, and his diagnosis.

You can't change the past. You can only change the future. You did the best you could. Feeling guilty only keeps you in the past. Yes, you feel sadness and disappointment about Steve getting prostate cancer. You would be wise to spend time processing your lingering grief over this situation.

Please consider setting aside some time to feel in your body where you store this pain. Schedule an appointment with Sherry to have her assist you in releasing the unhealthy cellular memory and journal about the life you miss.

Then commit to living in the present, consciously aware of your actions that create your future. Make sure you create the future you desire.

I love you, Cindie

Letting Love and Compassion Come Through

Increasing the love in my life holds more of a priority for me now than ever before. I found that my heart shut down during the challenging time of Steve's cancer and my mom's Alzheimer's diagnosis. I couldn't love very deeply. I felt wounded, unable to open my heart because it hurt so much.

Working with one of my teachers, Mother Pearl, I talked with her about my specific situation, and she assisted me in reopening my heart. Through just a few phone calls and in-person sessions, her energy and perspective guided me to feeling love again. With her kind, nurturing voice, she said, "Cindie, you have been given an opportunity to learn from these experiences, allowing you to teach and share techniques with others to reduce their pain." She added, "Learning how to love is the most important lesson we can learn, and learning it through hardships provides you with a reservoir of strength and courage. Your heart isn't broken, dear Cindie. It's cracking open." Relearning how to love, with Mother Pearl's assistance, allowed my heart to reveal itself in new ways.

As we love ourselves more, we can love others more, especially our men, who may greatly value our love to assist with *their* healing process. We can allow this love to freely flow from our heart to people all around us, boosting their energy and their spirits.

With the help of this teacher, I also found the capacity to bring more compassion to the world. I knew this would help me develop my feminine qualities, so I started looking at situations differently. Stepping into Steve's shoes and seeing things from his perspective, I can feel kinder toward him, especially when I'm not happy with our relationship.

I also discovered the importance of learning compassion for myself. Transforming a negative thought about myself with the words "I love you, Cindie" allows me to keep my love flowing. In addition, giving my body enough rest is a compassionate act I didn't used to allow myself. As I feel more rested, I'm able to feel more compassion, love for myself, and love for others.

Taking Responsibility for Oneself

Often, I feel the burden of other people weighing me down and causing tension in my shoulders. I still need to learn ways to let people live their own lives *their* way. When I do this, I can live *my* own life and not let anyone take responsibility for *me*. This way of thinking creates a sense of freedom in my life.

With my newfound freedom, though, came the realization that I am responsible for my own happiness or unhappiness, for choosing to survive or thrive. It also means I'm the only one who can make choices for my life. Steve can't make choices for me nor can anyone else.

I know also that I can't force Steve to do anything. I can suggest, encourage, insist, or plead for my husband to take specific actions, but in the end, I can only support him with his process. He is responsible for himself, just as I am responsible for myself. I used to believe I knew what was best for Steve, but I don't—as much as I dislike that idea.

It's apparent that releasing control continues to be a life lesson for me. I remind myself to put the word "surrender" into my vocabulary, something I couldn't do before. I used to view surrender as weak; now I see how it takes incredible strength to surrender and let go of controlling situations.

For example, if I don't believe Steve is recovering from prostate cancer fast enough, I must let go, providing him the opportunity to live his own life. No amount of nagging or angry words can change him. If he doesn't do what I think he must do to address his issues, I can't make him.

In fact, learning to take responsibility for myself causes me to learn to trust myself more. As I trust myself more, I find myself trusting more in others, knowing that each individual must take his or her own journey through life.

At some point, I came to this conclusion: Making choices about *my* life is what I can do. I can choose to stay unhappy in the marriage or decide to change something about my situation. If I can't find a way to be happy in my marriage with Steve, I can either choose to stay and accept the situation, or I can leave the marriage.

I don't intend this to sound threatening. Rather, it's an example of one way I learned how to thrive. A while back, I blamed Steve for our marriage not bringing me happiness. Living through the prostate cancer experience, I discovered that my happiness has to be generated within me. I decided not to live like a victim—not to give away my power but to keep it close as I make healthy choices in my life.

Fortunately, what I discovered on this journey allows my marriage to thrive after prostate cancer and releasing the control I thought I had over Steve has allowed him to thrive as well. What a win-win-win experience for me, for Steve, and for our marriage.

CHAPTER 4

THRIVING SPIRITUALLY

FOR ME, THE PATH TO thriving spiritually after prostate cancer means I am at peace. I feel centered and whole, connected with something much greater than I am.

I use the term Higher Power to describe a place or an entity I suggest connecting with to thrive after prostate cancer. Please substitute the name of your choice: God, Spirit, Universe, Source, All That Is, or something else that works for you.

Even if you don't believe in a Higher Power, please continue reading. The path to healing can follow whatever belief system rings true for you. Many paths exist to lead you to a life that thrives.

Connecting with All That Is

I grew up in the Southern Baptist faith. When the members of our church rejected my mother after her divorce, I became disillusioned with the whole concept of God and religion. It took me a long time to realize that my issues dealt with religion, not with God or a Higher Power. I sensed my connection with an entity much bigger than I am, yet something that's also part of me. Based on books that influenced me, I called it All That Is.

I searched for ways to talk with Mom and ease her fears, discovering that it helped to speak her language. After so many years of avoiding the word God, it took my mom's Alzheimer's diagnosis for me to become comfortable saying it. Even though she experienced rejection from the church, her beliefs and faith in God remained steadfast. Mom has found another church that accepted her, divorce and all. Amazingly, she still teaches Sunday school there, despite her disease.

It makes a tremendous difference to her when I mention God. It brings her peace during the frightening times she experiences, knowing her mind doesn't work the way it used to. After I decided to speak a more religious language to assist my mother, my openness to the benefit of religion expanded. In the process, it challenged my hurt feelings and long-standing grudge against religion.

Several years ago, I met an individual whose understanding of the Bible continues to astound me. She lives a life of providing gifts to everyone she meets. Her wisdom comes from her belief in God, her prayers, and her grounding in the teachings of the Bible. I enjoy listening to her and asking her questions, and I often find a great deal of similarity in our beliefs.

While my early path included Christian teachings, over the years I gravitated to studying Eastern beliefs and philosophies. I believe God lies within each one of us, connecting us to each other. The broad concept of All That Is still rings true for me.

I honor everyone's individual beliefs and enjoy conversations that explore spiritual topics. I especially like to discuss differing beliefs and then discover what we share in common. (As you read this section, please think of it in a way that's personal for you. Substitute your beliefs as required, allowing you to bring more peace into your life.)

Turning to Meditation and/or Prayer

The major difference between prayer and meditation is that prayer involves words and intention, or speaking to God, while meditation involves stilling the mind, listening to God, or experiencing deep peace. However, many find that prayer *takes them* to this space of peace and quiet, that space in which they can hear God speaking to them with comforting words. Interestingly, *Amazon.com* lists three times the number of books that teach "prayer" compared to those teaching "meditation."

Regardless of your beliefs, a daily practice of meditation will move you forward on your journey and keep you thriving. Some people consider prayers to be meditation; others meditate through certain types of activities, such as walking, gardening, cleaning; still others meditate by becoming still and quieting the mind and body.

For me, a daily practice of meditation gives me time to contemplate, create intentions for my day, and listen to my inner voice, my Higher Power. I started meditating in the 1980s after a partner in the big accounting firm I had joined shared a chilling message with me. I had met this man briefly right after college when I traveled through Europe and met with partners of the firm. In Belgium, we shared a delightful multi-course lunch. Although I don't recall his name, he had a tremendous impact on my life. To this day, I often send him grateful thoughts.

About two years after our first meeting, I saw this man at a training session. He took me aside and told me I wasn't the relaxed young woman he had met in Belgium. Instead, he saw a stressed out, unhealthy woman, and he expressed concern for my well-being. Then he assured me that working as a CPA would only become more challenging, and that I needed to find a way to reduce my tension immediately. He frightened me so much with his observation of how much I had changed that I immediately followed his advice. I bought a short book by Herbert Benson, MD titled *The Relaxation Response* and began a regular practice of meditation to reduce my stress.

Most of the time since then, I've started my day with meditation. I use a method taught by Deepak Chopra, MD, the "ah" meditation offered by Dr. Wayne Dyer, and guided meditations from Learning Strategies Corporation that incorporate Holosync® technology. (See Resources section.)

When Steve and I met, he mentioned his desire to learn how to meditate. Over a Thanksgiving holiday in Sedona one year, Steve learned Dr. Chopra's primordial sound meditation method, which I had previously learned at The Chopra Center.

Benefits of Meditation

Many people say they can't sit still long enough to meditate or they tried and couldn't get their mind to stop chattering. If meditation speaks to you, find a teacher and/or a book to help you learn, or just sit quietly, observing your breath. Meditation helps bring you into balance physically, emotionally, and mentally. It allows you to think more clearly, make better choices, and reduce stress. It also lowers blood pressure and increases energy.

For me, hiking by myself is a form of meditation. Some people find themselves in a meditative state when they cook, garden, run, or walk. I suggest you do something that allows your mind to

---

disengage and stop chattering—an activity that brings you peace and the ability to hear your inner voice.

Regardless of the method you choose to create peace in your life, discover one that works for you. As you enhance your practice, your inner voice/God's voice/intuition will become more prominent, allowing you to hear messages that help you create a thriving life.

Circle Drawing and Journaling

Earlier, I mentioned expanding the awareness of our five senses. We can also expand our sixth sense, our intuition, to bring insights to our healing process. Creating circle drawings and journaling are two ways to connect with our inner voices and quiet our minds.

Circle Drawing

Making circle drawings allows us to expand our knowledge, exploring a concept and digging deeper into a question to obtain new information. Often, they lead us to surprises.

I use circle drawings to answer questions and discover information that doesn't come easily to me. They also help me hear what my right brain—my creative side—wants to say, keeping my left brain—my analytical side—out of the way. I also use this technique to build on an idea, continuing to search for that next right answer.

To do a circle drawing, I start with a blank piece of paper, preferably one without lines. In the middle of the page, I draw a big circle and write a question inside it. I then allow answers to the question to come through me via my right brain. I like to do circle drawings at my kitchen table where I have a view of Camelback Mountain. To relax before I start, I close my eyes and take several deep breaths. I like to get into a meditative state, which reduces unrelated thoughts flashing through my mind. While that is an ideal situation for me, I've obtained answers from doing circle drawings on an airplane and in a crowded classroom.

I draw a line from the main circle, put a circle at the end of it, and insert my first answer to the question. The next answer may be on a completely different topic, so I draw another line from the main circle and insert the answer there. If my next answer is related to the second answer, I draw a line from that second circle, add another circle, and insert my answer. I continue this process for about 10 minutes.

What are the keys to doing this technique? Writing fast and keeping my left brain out of the way. (Some people find writing with their non-dominant hand further connects them with their right brain and their heart.) I don't question my answers as I write; I only view them with curiosity, keenly interested to discover the next answer.

Too often, especially when we live in survival mode, we over-think everything. Our left brain takes over, reducing access to our heart and other ways to understand how to best move forward. In effect, circle drawing gives the left brain a chance to take a relaxing vacation.

Through circle drawings, I discovered what sexual fulfillment means to me. I also learned what thriving after prostate cancer looks like. In both cases, answers came through me that I hadn't considered before and opened up entirely new paths for me to follow.

When I drew a big circle on a blank piece of paper and wrote the question, "What is sexual fulfillment?" my answers helped me realize it wasn't all about orgasms or sexual intercourse. Sexual fulfillment connects me with my Higher Power, with feelings of peace and oneness.

See part of my circle drawing as an example.

May 29, 2010

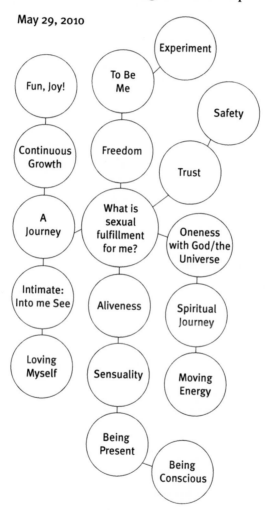

This activity told me my former definition of sexual fulfillment didn't ring true. By using the circle drawing technique, I discovered I could reach sexual fulfillment by myself; I didn't require a partner. Then I saw I could reach a *different* level of sexual fulfillment with a partner, and the circle drawing gave me insights for improving my relationship with Steve to become more sexually fulfilled. This discovery helped me gain power and inspired me to take responsibility for my own fulfillment.

Every day, I realize that as my sexual fulfillment expands, I feel more compassionate toward Steve and become a better partner for him. I know how to better support him in his own process of gaining sexual fulfillment. After creating my circle drawing, I asked him for his definition of sexual fulfillment so I could better understand his desires and support his healing process. While he didn't actually do a circle drawing, he defined sexual fulfillment for him as emotional closeness, physical intimacy, and mental intensity. He also included words like trust, passion, vulnerability, oneness, and excitement in his definition.

Journaling

Amazingly, on *Amazon.com*, the number of books about journaling equals the number of books on meditation and prayer combined! Yes, you can choose from more than 1,300 books to help you learn how to journal. Some people use Julia Cameron's process of writing Morning Pages as described in her book, *The Artist's Way*. Others take classes to learn how to journal or just start writing. You can easily find information on journaling to help you on your journey.

Periodically, I give myself the treat of buying a new journal. Because journaling remains popular, I find a variety of covers, sizes, and colors. I also buy journals on my travels, providing me with another special memory of my trip. In the unlikely event that I don't have a journal on hand, I just use a pad of paper or the computer to write down my thoughts and feelings—and enjoy the insights that come up.

Whether I find answers to questions from circle drawings, journaling, or some other method, I'm generally astonished at what comes through. Often the insights I receive bring me much more than I imagined possible—and many times more than one helpful answer.

Try These for Yourself!

If circle drawing or journaling appeals to you, take time to try them out. They will assist your process of discovery, understanding, and growth. Recognize that the journey to thriving after prostate cancer provides unique opportunities for each woman. Identifying *exactly* what thriving means becomes your personal road map.

Living with Purpose and Passion

Thriving after prostate cancer requires finding inspiration in our lives. This also assists our man with his healing and regaining passion and purpose in his life. When we live our passion, we invite our man to participate in it. It might even help him find his own purpose after prostate cancer.

Find Your Passionate Calling

Your mate's prostate cancer diagnosis could coincide with the time in your life when your children leave home, or when you start welcoming grandchildren into your family. One or both of you may be retired and suddenly finding yourself with lots of free time. I invite

---

you to use this time to find your passionate calling—that next part of life that will bring you meaning.

Perhaps your life up to this time revolved around caring for others. Once your man becomes healthy again, give yourself the gift of focusing on you. To begin, you may want to create a list of projects and areas to explore.

If you don't know where to start, look back at your childhood to discover what activities thrilled you back then. What might bring you meaning now? Perhaps you could relearn how to play that musical instrument or take a painting class, make jewelry, take cooking lessons, or learn a foreign language. What sounds like fun to you?

Most men will support their women in these endeavors. After all, "When Momma's happy, everyone's happy." Use the request format to communicate your desire to explore your passionate calling to your man. Here's what that conversation might look like:

"Steve, may I disturb you for just a minute? I want to arrange a time to talk about starting an activity that means a lot to me."

"The golf tournament is almost over. Let's talk later this afternoon."

Later . . .

"Did you enjoy watching the golf tournament, Steve? What I want to talk about reminds me of the golfers and how many of them had a dream of playing professional golf since they were kids. In my case, I'd like to attend a writing retreat and write a book. I've wanted to do this since I was a little girl."

"What would you write about, where's the retreat, and can I go with you?"

"There's a five-day writing retreat in Sedona next March. The advertising claims almost everyone who attends the retreat finishes a book. I'd like to give it a try. I'm not sure what I'd write about. I can figure that out before the retreat. I guess you could go along, although I'll be at the retreat most of the day and some evenings. Would you support me in attending?"

"What would I need to do?"

"Support my time away and my preparation time. I understand there's homework to do before the retreat. There's also technology involved, so you could help me get into the retreat website and make sure my computer will work at the retreat."

"So you'd like me to make sure you have the technology you need? You'll also be away from home and need to spend time preparing before you go."

"Yes. Are you willing to support me with this?"

"Yes. It sounds like this would make you really happy."

"It would be a dream come true. Thank you for helping me fulfill my childhood fantasy of writing a book."

Take time to find inspiration in the post-prostate cancer part of your life. Having fun and living a life that excites you will cause you and your man to thrive.

Creating a Special Space in Your Home

Whether you start a new endeavor or continue projects already in place, make sure to create a special space in your home just for you. You may hear about making sure a man has his "cave" in a home. Many people assume this means the rest of the house belongs to the woman. I suggest you create your own cave, a special place in your home, which belongs just to you. Find a corner of your home that can become your spiritual home or space.

You can read, pray, cry, journal, and/or rejuvenate in your special space. I invite you to decorate it in a way that brings you joy and peace. Add books, statues, cards, artwork, incense, and flowers—anything that causes you to smile. Make sure you can breathe deeply and feel completely safe in your space. As you know, prostate cancer can cause a lot of fear and angst, so create a place that will augment your healing process.

Use the feedback format to make sure your man supports you in creating your space. Ask him to help, letting him know what this space provides for you. Make sure he knows your intention to rejuvenate yourself, not to avoid him or escape from him. Request that he leave you alone when you spend time there for that purpose. Make sure he knows not to ask for your help to find the car keys or dig up something in the refrigerator. As you ask your man to help you set aside time for yourself, also ask him to protect that space for you and keep you safe there.

Feng Shui

The concept of feng shui is said to improve the energy of an environment based on the arrangement of objects and other physical adjustments. It's important to use its principles to make sure the energy feels right in that space. To learn more about feng shui, explore these ancient Chinese principles of design to facilitate positive energy.

Many women naturally know how to create an inviting home. They love spending time updating and changing the look of their space. If you, like me, don't have this knack or desire to learn, feng shui can help. Many different methods of feng shui exist; accessing books and consultants will get you started.

Feng shui principles have helped me create a home that feels comfortable and looks pleasing to the eye. I'm able to use colors and place items in ways that create certain effects and support certain goals. When I feel good about my home, my energy flows freely. I know Steve and I will feel that energy and live a healthier, happier life in this supportive space.

Looking for the Gifts

As Steve and I continue to assist people in their recovery from prostate cancer, people say "you are really turning lemons into lemonade." I value that observation and look for ways to use my prostate cancer experience to help others lead happier lives.

I love reading messages from the media star Oprah Winfrey because her knack for finding the gift in every experience inspires me. I appreciate all reminders to look for what each situation in life brings me, although I admit to struggling at times to find the gifts from my mom's Alzheimer's disease.

That said, my experience with Steve's healing process has allowed me to more fully engage with my mom's situation, bringing more patience and compassion into her life and providing more resources for her well-being. I can love her more unconditionally now than I did before, partially due to my own views of spirituality and mortality that have developed over this period. Perhaps one of my gifts from her disease is the opportunity to use what I've learned and deepen my skills.

As time goes by, I can look back and more easily find the gifts. When I perceive a recent event in my life as "bad," I can't find many gifts. But as time goes by and I see all that transpired around the event, many gifts appear. Time does help me heal.

Prostate cancer gave me a husband with better eating habits. (Yes, Steve's diagnosis scared him in ways that only a person can understand who experiences a close brush with death.) After his diagnosis, he immediately started improving his diet. He even eliminated some foods he had enjoyed most of his life, including red meat and milk, and started eating more vegetables, drinking pomegranate juice and selecting organic products.

Another gift I received from prostate cancer included a chance to address many of my own issues by finding everything *unlike love* in my being. Sometimes looking at my dark side is painful. As I face my issues, though, I find that much of my joy in life comes from personal growth. That means I can handle challenges more easily than before because of the skills I learned as a prostate cancer survivor.

Steve and I definitely enjoy a better sex life and a stronger marriage than we did before prostate cancer. Now that we don't just focus on intercourse and orgasms to bring us sexual

---

Become an Ambassador and Educator

As you ask more questions after prostate cancer, you might become an ambassador to encourage men to get tested regularly and obtain treatment, if required. I urge you to become an educator, encouraging healthy eating and stress reduction. Consider turning your experience into a gift that keeps on giving to others.

Prostate cancer can be the perfect teacher for finding gifts in every experience. Journaling or circle drawing may shed some light on this for you. Draw a big circle on a blank piece of paper with the question, "What gifts did my prostate cancer experience provide for me?" Then see what answers arise.

Whether you want to write about your experience, work in a cancer recovery center, or encourage men to get tested on a regular basis, reframing your prostate cancer as a gift can speed you toward living a life that thrives.

---

pleasure, the menu of options to expand our lovemaking has grown. Also, our intimacy and ability to talk about all topics has greatly increased. Our conversations these days bring me much more joy than before our prostate cancer journey.

I've become a resource for the many people in my life who receive a prostate cancer diagnosis or who know a person in their life with prostate cancer. While I never set out to play this role, I'm grateful to answer questions and provide comfort to others. You can find my contact information at *www.SolutionsForIntimacy.com.*

Facing Our Mortality—and Immortality

Once a woman hears the prostate cancer diagnosis about a man she loves, a natural follow-up question deals with his mortality. From there, a woman then thinks about her own mortality. When Steve received his diagnosis, I pondered what my life would look like if I lost him to death.

Depending on your relationship with the man, your thoughts will take different paths. If your dad receives the diagnosis, you wonder how it will feel to lose a parent. If your brother receives the news, you think about his children losing a father or his wife losing her husband. If your mate ends up with prostate cancer, you wonder about your financial security or how you can exist on your own without his helping hand.

I was concerned about Steve's lack of conversation after his diagnosis. More than once, I'd asked, "Steve, ever since you received the diagnosis, you've been really quiet. Is there something you'd like to share with me?" After a long pause, he said, "I've been contemplating my own mortality." OMG! Up to that moment, I hadn't thought that Steve might *die*. I thought prostate cancer was relatively common and easy to treat.

He continued, "I've been thinking about how important relationships are to my life and wanting to make sure that special people in my life know how much I love them. I'm also wondering if my will needs updating."

"What else are you thinking about?" I asked with amazement. I had no idea Steve was experiencing these thoughts.

"Well, I'm gaining more satisfaction when I'm involved with day-to-day activities, enjoying it more when we laugh, and when I talk with Sean. I appreciate our travels together and when I make a difference for someone at work."

Once he shared these powerful thoughts with me, I started wondering about my own mortality. I wonder if special people in my life know how much I love them. Have I made amends with everyone in my life? Does my will need updating? I made a commitment to live each day even more fully than before.

Questioning myself about life after death caused me to further deepen my spiritual understanding of the afterlife. I read books and talked with various teachers about their beliefs. For me, I concluded that death is a transition from the physical body and that the soul lives on. For you, your exploring may come in the form of going back to church, talking with religious experts, and praying a lot.

Often, our beliefs about what happens after death can provide comfort. My belief that our spirits continue to live allowed me to know that Steve would "go on," as sung by Celine Dion in the song "My Heart Will Go On" from the movie *Titanic*. The opening lines of the song are highly meaningful to me: *Every night in my dreams, I see you, I feel you. That is how I know you go on.* I believe that when he departs from the physical world, he will continue participating in my life in another form.

Many people believe those who die will go to heaven to live with God, and that heaven provides a much better place to live than Earth. Although this belief doesn't take away the sadness and the hole that exists from losing a loved one, it can bring a measure of comfort.

Clear the Air about Death

Talk with your man or with someone else about your deaths. Until this conversation happens, often the thought of death becomes an elephant in the room and remains on people's minds. Clear the air about this topic, no matter how long ago your man received his diagnosis. If you don't want to bring up the topic of cancer, consider using the need to revise your will to start the conversation. You must talk about the end of life in order to properly plan for your family. Doing so will bring you much peace.

Death often brings feelings of fear to the surface. Talking about the future and planning for that time provides more knowledge to help dissipate the fear. Steve and I found our prostate cancer experience originally caused us to drift apart. As we began to look at the various parts of our relationship and at ourselves, our connection to each other became stronger than before. Our love deepened, causing us to feel grateful for this disease that propelled us into discovering how to live a life that thrives.

I wish that for you, too.

WHAT I WOULD DO DIFFERENTLY

OFTEN PEOPLE ASK what I would do differently if I could restart this journey.

First, I would have found ways to improve my physical relationship with Steve much sooner than I did. I settled for the notion of being grateful that Steve is alive. In effect, I accepted our relationship as a good friendship without the passion that enhances a great marriage.

Second, I would have supported Steve using the ErecAid® vacuum therapy system he purchased soon after surgery. We call it "the pump." It's a battery-operated device that assists Steve in achieving an erection quickly without the side effects of drug therapy. I could have incorporated the pump into our intimacy sessions sooner, making the experience more playful and fun.

Third, I would have encouraged Steve to open up about his prostate cancer earlier, thus allowing me to talk about it with more people. Rather than hiding the situation, we both could have allowed others to help us much sooner after his surgery.

Solutions for Intimacy

Perhaps reading about my experience will provide you with inspiration to improve your life. You can probably add to this list, based on your own lessons learned.

Join me on *www.SolutionsForIntimacy.com* to continue the conversation and assist one another in our healing. Share the gifts you found from your prostate cancer experience, ask questions, and provide answers to others. Together we can thrive after prostate cancer!

A New Diagnosis

After I began addressing comments from Barbara McNichol's first round of edits, Steve called me at work following an appointment with a neurologist. "Cindie, the doctor diagnosed me with Parkinson's disease. He says it's not life-threatening."

When I got home that evening, we held each other closely, breathing together. Steve then said, "Please tell anyone you want about my diagnosis. Until I read your book, I had no idea how difficult it was for you not to share my prostate cancer diagnosis and surgery. I don't want you to go through that again. Also, we'll do a better job this time. I'll communicate more, and we're going to approach this diagnosis in an entirely different way."

In the two weeks since Steve called with this news, I've cycled through the grieving process multiple times. My anger came swiftly, followed by a denial of the diagnosis and a bargaining that, if the diagnosis were accurate, "it wouldn't be so bad."

The sadness, the tears, the fear, and the depression arrived frequently and sometimes without warning. I've cycled in and out of acceptance several times. Thankfully, I live there most of the time right now.

Believe me, it has helped to share this news with friends. One person connected us with an expert in the field so Steve could schedule an appointment with him for a second opinion. Another provided diet and exercise recommendations; others shared their resources and a sense of humor.

My morning meditations provide a guaranteed place of peace, and I'm using my knowledge about men to communicate better with Steve. I'm also bringing more of my feminine energy to our life this time, allowing creativity to flow more freely. I'm also allowing Steve to take the lead.

I've already found a gift—that is, affirmation that the techniques in this guide work! By gaining knowledge, I am eliminating my fear. By staying present, I take each day as it arrives. I breathe deeply, dance ecstatically, and make love with enthusiasm.

Although I wasn't planning to practice what I wrote about so soon, I'm grateful to have this guide at hand to help me thrive. I hope that you are, too.

ACKNOWLEDGMENTS

WRITING GIVES ME many gifts—the gift of self-discovery, the gift of understanding the concepts in this guide better, and of course, the gift of thriving after prostate cancer.

With my husband, Steve Frohman, at my side, I learned about intimacy. As with other endeavors, I looked within and became intimate with myself before I could become intimate with him. He was required to do the same, and I marvel at his courage and strength, as he continues to uncover new layers of himself.

As I typically do when learning new skills, I found the best resources available to assist me. Sherry Anshara, QuantumPathic® Center of Consciousness, assisted me to transform my life from one of reactivity and limited beliefs, to one of conscious responses and unlimited possibilities. Albert Gaulden and the Sedona Intensive team supported me as I dissected events in my life, allowing me to discover reasons for the unhealthy patterns and teaching me ways to break them.

My ongoing support team assists me in staying healthy, both inside and out. Kathleen, Sharon, Rachelle, Sandy, Mother Pearl, Jivana, Andrea, Terri, Adell, Pat, Corinne, and Dan listen without judgment and love me unconditionally. Dr. Larry Bans supports Steve's health, which in turn supports me.

I started working with writing coach Tom Bird five years ago. This is the fourth book I've written, the first to be published, and Tom has walked with me along this path that included several life-changing events. Writing brings up emotional issues for me, and I'm grateful for his wise counsel during challenging times.

Barbara McNichol edited this book and suggested the subtitle. I knew I wanted to work with her from the first time I met her. Her professionalism, enjoyment of her craft, and many talents created a guide for you that's become more fun to read with each review.

I love working with the Arizona Society of CPAs where I get to partner with a tremendous staff and fantastic volunteers. I'm fortunate to count many of these people as close friends and appreciate how they care about me and my path of self-discovery. Adela, Cynthia, Heidi, Jena, José, Mary, Patty, and Traci traveled many steps with me along the way. Peggy, Dan, Julie, Ken and Nancy, David, George, Rufus, Bill, Rick, and Mark shared hours of their lives with me.

While I'm new with my Vistage CEO group, the members embrace me and my different way of looking at matters. Group leader Conrad holds an important space for me to learn about myself while group member Keith provides legal guidance and connections.

My small family is a big part of my life. My mother, Pat Howell, also provided me the opportunity to look inside myself as I took on a new role after her diagnosis with Alzheimer's disease three years ago. My sister Beth Brock and her husband Bob Greenawalt partner with me in those efforts. They share my love of travel and of supporting women and the environment.

Andrea Aker and Beth Cochran quickly understood how Steve and I intend to assist others live sexually fulfilled lives. Their expertise in design, writing, marketing, and technology launched Solutions for Intimacy and took The Personal Approach to new levels.

Life is a gift. I'm grateful to be alive and grateful to the many people who support me in creating a life that *thrives*.

RESOURCES FOR MOVING FROM SURVIVING TO THRIVING

Sherry Anshara, QuantumPathic® Center of Consciousness, *www.quantumpathic.com*

Anyone interested in personal growth would benefit from spending time with Sherry. She and her team quickly and effortlessly get to the heart of the matter, transforming the lives of those fortunate enough to experience the QuantumPathic® Energy Method in person or by phone.

Larry Bans, MD, Prostate Solutions of Arizona, *www.psa.md*

Dr. Bans is Steve's urologist. During surgery, he took a break to talk with me. After he left, a person in the waiting area asked if the doctor was a good friend of mine. I said, no, I had only met him a few times. That's just who Dr. Bans is—an expert surgeon, and one of the most compassionate, caring, and open-minded medical professionals I have ever met.

Tom Bird, writing coach extraordinaire, *www.writeyourbookin8days.com*

Whether you've ever wanted to write a book or not, do yourself a favor—attend one of Tom's writing retreats. Even if your book never gets published, you will learn so much about yourself from his guidance to make the investment worth it.

Andrea Beaulieu, coach, storyteller, singer, *www.AndreaBeaulieu.com*

Andrea's the one who challenged me to change my story in a formative moment of my life one year ago. She's taught for the ASCPA and helped Steve tell his story. Her authentic voice rings loudly for all who are fortunate to work with her.

Feng Shui with Marie Diamond, *www.MarieDiamond.com*

This feng shui expert offers truly unique ways of incorporating feng shui principles into your home and office. Marie helped me "cure" a section of our home that never felt safe to me. You can also find her material at *www .LearningStrategies.com.*

Albert Gaulden, founder, The Sedona Intensive, *www.SedonaIntensive.com*

Albert, Scott, and their team continue to influence the lives of their students in profound ways. To put your life into overdrive, read Albert's book, *You're Not Who You Think You Are,* have him do an astrological reading, and participate in an Intensive.

Kathleen Gramzay, massage therapist,
www.kneadforbalance.com

Keeping my body free of tension and moving easily is what Kathleen does with Kinessage® Massage Through Movement. While I'm on her massage table, she allows me to process my thoughts and questions with ease.

Gay and Katie Hendricks, authors, *Conscious Breathing* (and others), *www.hendricks.com*

When I made a resolution that my marriage to Steve would last, I began reading books by this amazing couple. Their material—the best I found on relationship-building—works! I continue to learn from the Henricks' amusing examples and online resources, and I get inspiration from their passion.

Cindie Hubiak and Steve Frohman,
www.SolutionsForIntimacy.com

We assist others to thrive after prostate cancer by looking at sex in a whole new way. See our website and blog for more resources.

Mother Pearl Justice, relationship oracle
MotherPearl@verizon.net

There can't be many more loving people in this world than Mother Pearl. Hearing her voice on the phone, receiving a hug, and benefiting from her insights have propelled me and Steve forward through many pivotal points in our marriage.

Dr. Sharon Lamm-Hartman, coach,
www.insideoutlearninginc.com

Dr. Sharon guided me through her passionate calling process, allowing me to understand my gifts and life purpose. Her teaching and coaching has produced extraordinary results for me, my staff members, and CPA volunteers.

Learning Strategies Corporation,
www.LearningStrategies.com

This is one of the leading human potential organizations around. I use its meditations almost daily. I've gained powerful insights from their conferences and own almost everything they have produced. To put a fire into your relationship, use its *Creating Sparks* Paraliminal.

Mary J. Lore, author and teacher,
www.ManagingThought.com

I met Mary when she taught a program for leaders of the ASCPA where I work. I discovered that the techniques in her book, *Managing Thought,* provide a road map to self-awareness, improved creativity, and living life full of gratitude.

Sandy Lutrin, N.D., *www.doctorlutrin.com*

Dr. Lutrin supported Steve and me through his prostate cancer diagnosis, referred us to the Tantrika, has helped my hormones stay balanced during perimenopause, and is a key member of our Parkinson's disease team.

Rachelle Marmor, acupuncturist,
www.arizona-acupuncture.com

Whenever I ask Rachelle whether acupuncture can provide relief for a certain condition, she answers yes. And she's right. Her dedication to her craft, her devotion to helping others live a pain-free life, and her work in the international community is admirable.

Sarah McLean, meditation instructor,
www.SedonaMeditation.com

Steve took a meditation class from Sarah about 10 years ago. Since then, we've followed Sarah's skyrocketing career as she helps others reduce stress and improve health through her meditation instruction.

Barbara McNichol, editor, *www.BarbaraMcNichol.com*

I had worked with three editors on other books before hiring Barbara. I didn't know what real editing was all about until I received my manuscript back from her the first time. My words came alive and started to sing from her first draft.

Men/relationship resources:

Susie and Otto Collins, relationship/life success coaches,
www.collinspartners.com

The Collins' material is practical, fun to read, and easy to implement.

Bob Grant, LPC, The Relationship Doctor,
www.relationshipheadquarters.com

Bob helped me learn what would cause Steve to adore me. I especially liked his program "What Husbands Can't Resist."

PAX programs, *www.understandmen.com*

Of all the organizations I worked with, Steve says this has had the most positive impact on my behavior in our relationship. And he has supported me in attending almost every PAX program offered.

Neti Pot, *http://sinucleanse.com*

My neti pot and I go everywhere together. Another source for neti pots is:

www.webmd.com/allergies/sinus-pain-pressure-9/neti-pots

Dr. Christiane Northrup, author, visionary pioneer, *www.drnorthrup.com*

Dr. Northrup's book, *The Secret Pleasures of Menopause,* provides a wealth of information for women on their own health and the well-being of their intimate relationship.

Prostate cancer books for men and couples (available at *amazon.com* and other places):

Intimacy with Impotence and *The Lovin' Ain't Over* by Ralph and Barbara Alterowitz

Making Love Again by Virginia and Keith Laken

The Prostate Storm by Steve Vogel

Tantrika and other Tantra resources:

Jivana Kennedy, Tantrika, *www.TantricHealingTouch.com*

Jivana's intuition, deep knowledge, and care for Steve and me provided us with creative ways to increase our intimacy.

For a treasure chest of information, go to *www.tantra.com.*

Charles and Caroline Muir, *www.sourcetantra.com* **and** *www.divine-feminine.com*

These renowned Tantric teachers offer several ways to learn about conscious loving, including the following that are sure to educate and excite:

- *Secrets of Female Sexual Ecstasy,* DVD

- *Freeing the Female Orgasm,* audio book

- *Tantra: The Art of Conscious Loving,* hardcover or paperback

ABOUT THE AUTHOR

CINDIE HUBIAK has created successful relationships throughout her distinguished career as a CPA, CEO, human resources director, business manager, leader, mentor, and sexuality educator. International stints in Europe and Asia taught her the value of cross-cultural communication—a key in building meaningful relationships. As she sees it, work life, play life, and home life are simply better when relationships thrive.

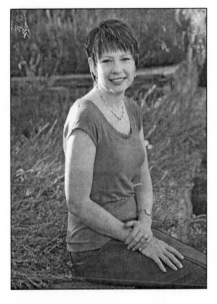

Suffering in silence after her husband Steve's prostate cancer diagnosis, she had to wake up to her deep-seated unhappiness. She sought remedies—not just for his disease but for their waning intimacy and her own emotional turmoil. Her earnest search led her to revitalize her relationship with Steve and emerge as a happy, sensual, sexual woman.

Whether it's through her mentoring, her leadership, or her training skills, Cindie consistently strives to live her values. She loves to give to others as she builds relationships with family, friends, colleagues, and people in the community.

"Steve and Cindie are the right people at the right time. They have created an approach to sexual fulfillment after prostate disease that works."

—Dr. Sandy Lutrin, Phoenix, Arizona

SOLUTIONS FOR INTIMACY provides couples with the tools, resources, and knowledge to enjoy a sexually fulfilling life after prostate cancer.

Husband-and-wife team Steve Frohman and Cindie Hubiak founded the program following Steve's courageous battle with prostate cancer. Although he beat the disease, concern about reviving their sex life hovered over the couple like a dark cloud. They ultimately tackled all the barriers to intimacy through their focus on learning more, experimenting more, and—most of all—loving more.

To develop their Solutions for Intimacy program, Steve and Cindie assembled a team of top-notch experts spanning multiple facets of health and wellness. Their goal? To help couples get to the root issues of their intimacy struggles and enable them to thrive. They use a methodology called The Personal Approach—Living a Sexually Fulfilling Life after Prostate Disease. Tailored to a couple's uniqueness, it addresses the physical, emotional, mental, and spiritual aspects of intimacy. For detailed information, visit *www.SolutionsForIntimacy.com*.

CPSIA information can be obtained at www.ICGtesting.com
Printed in the USA
LVOW121641080213

319318LV00005B/707/P